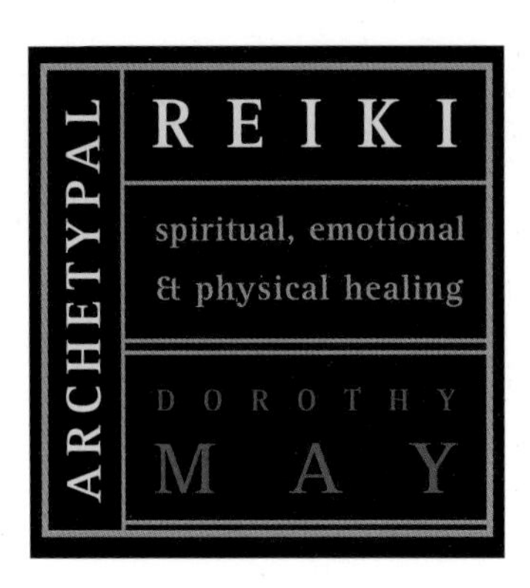
ARCHETYPAL
REIKI
spiritual, emotional
& physical healing
DOROTHY
MAY

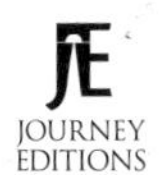
JOURNEY
EDITIONS

First published in 2000 by Journey Editions, an imprint of Periplus Editions (HK) Ltd.,
with editorial offices at 153 Milk Street, Boston, Massachusetts, 02109.

Library of Congress Cataloging-in-Publication Data

May, Dorothy
Archetypal Reiki : book and cards for spiritual, emotional, and physical healing / Dorothy May. -- 1st ed
p. cm.
ISBN 1-885203-90-X (pb)
1. Reiki (Healing system) 2. Mental healing. I. Title.
RZ403.R45M29 2000
615.8'52--dc21 99-40403
CIP

Distributed by

USA
Tuttle Publishing
Distribution Center
Airport Industrial Park
364 Innovation Drive
North Clarendon, VT
05759-9436
Tel: (802) 773-8930
Tel: (800) 526-2778

JAPAN
Tuttle Shuppan
RK Building, 2nd Floor
2-13-10 Shimo-Meguro, Meguro-Ku
Tokyo 153 0064
TEL: (03) 5437-0171
FAX: (03) 5437-0755

CANADA
Raincoast Books
8680 Cambie Street
Vancouver, British Columbia V6P 6M9
Tel: (604) 323-7100
Fax: (604) 323-2600

SOUTHEAST ASIA
Berkeley Books Pte Ltd
5 Little Road #08-01
Singapore 536983
Tel: (65) 280-1330
Fax: (65) 280-6290

This book is sold only as part of *Archetypal Reiki*. It is not to be sold seperately.

Art Direction & design: Michele Wetherbee, double-u-gee, Petaluma, California, U.S.A.
Original illustrations: © Nicholas Wilton, San Anselmo, California, U.S.A.
Produced by Regent Publishing Services
Printed in Hong Kong

06 05 04 03 02 01 00 10 9 8 7 6 5 4 3 2 1

I dedicate this work to Dr. Carl Jung, father of the archetype; to Dr. Mikao Usui, founder of Reiki; and to the many Reiki Masters, Teachers, and Guides who have been with me from the beginning. Forever and now. I dedicate myself and my work to the Spirit of Healing Energy that flows through each of us.

I gratefully acknowledge
Dr. Kathleen W. FitzGerald and Laura Adams, Reiki Master-Teacher, for the loving energy it took to read and comment on my original manuscript. Thanks for the finger painting, too!
Steven May, Mary Wolf, and Katherine Bristow for their original inspirational artwork.
Chris Carlsen of The Creative Source for creating the original Archetypal Reiki brochure.
Cyndi Chekel, Steven May, Janet Mroczek, Adrienne Pearlman, and Kathy Sweeney for their loving support.
The Chicago Mentor Group for the Magic of Love.
Hal Bennett and Susan Sparrow, for being available.
Jan Johnson for smart decisions.

It takes a common vision to raise a child. It takes a common vision to raise a book. I thank the Voices from the past; the Sight from the future; the Wisdom from the now.

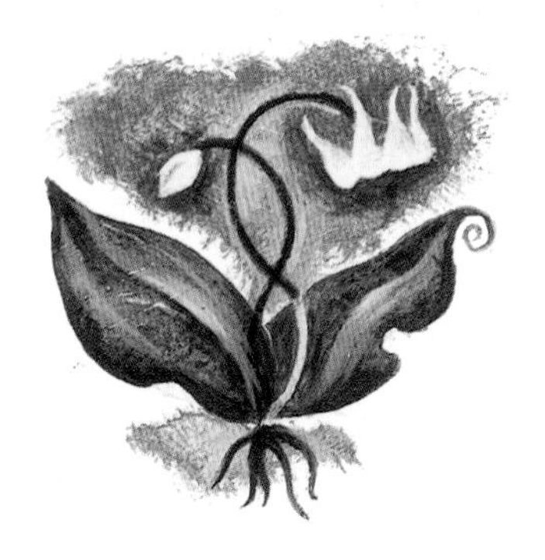

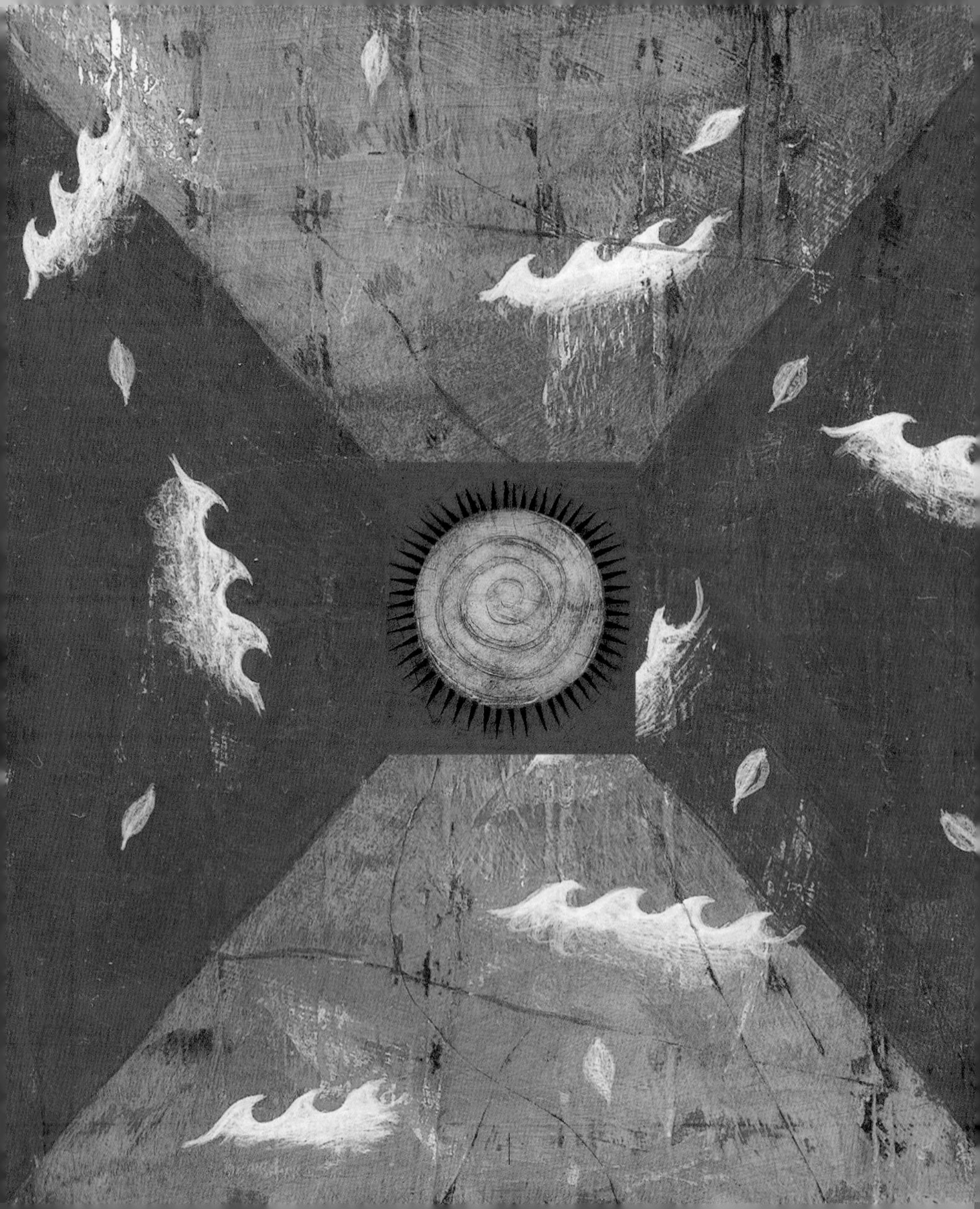

TABLE OF CONTENTS

This book is organized so it can be read from beginning to end and you can read it that way the first time. You may also use pieces of it, according to your inner knowing guidance.

Caveat.
I have here included the Reiki Japanese symbol names but not the actual symbols. The symbols are not secret but are sacred and will not work unless one has been attuned. To become a Reiki practitioner requires the proper ceremony of attunement by a Reiki Master-Teacher who has him/herself been attuned by a Master-Teacher. The Archetypal Reiki Card system is not a substitute for traditional Reiki attunement or Reiki energy healing.

Archetypal Reiki is in and of itself a spiritual path and a supplement to any spiritual practice. All of this material must be used with utmost respect and honor for the Spirit of Healing, which honors all traditions.

We must learn to offer the world a way of approach that honors both ego's desire to be holy and the soul's true delight at getting to be all too human. —Jacqueline Small

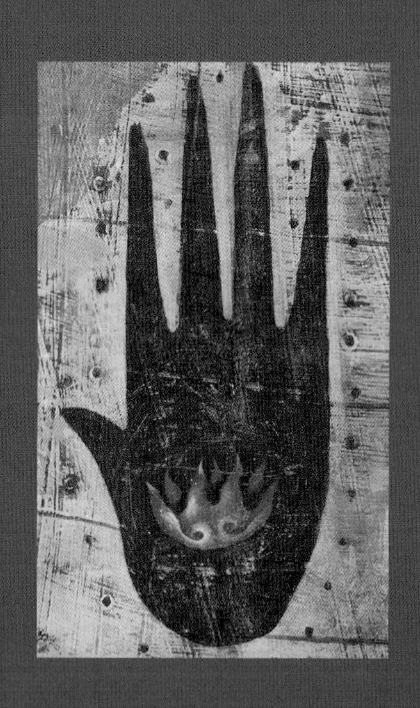

INTRODUCTION Reiki Healing & the Archetypal Reiki Cards

The system of healing we know as Reiki (pronounced ray-key) was rediscovered in the early part of the twentieth century by Japanese scholar and holy man Mikao Usui (me-ka-o you-soo-ee). Out of an interest in the healing methods of Jesus, Buddha, and other great healers, Dr. Usui searched all the known writings—Christian, ancient Japanese, Chinese—to find out how healing happened. He studied the ancient formulas and symbols of Tibet and found a formula in Sanskrit for healing. But neither he nor anyone else could actually perform the healings described in the formula.

In the early 1900s, he went to the Kuriyama Temple on the holy mountain Kuriyama in Kyoto, Japan, to seek spiritual answers. He stayed there in solitude, measuring time by placing twenty-one little stones on the ground and removing one each day. During this time, he read the sutras, chanted, meditated, and fasted. Nothing happened, though he had great faith.

As is often the case, it wasn't until the morning of the last day that his faith was rewarded. He saw a shining light moving toward him at great speed. It grew bigger and bigger as it got closer until he thought he was going to die when it hit him. Instead of killing him, the light hit him in the middle of the forehead. This was his spiritual awakening. Some say that he saw the colors of blue, white, and purple in the form of bubbles, and that in the bubbles were four Sanskrit symbols glowing in gold. When the enlightenment entered him, he felt full of strength and energy. On the way back down the mountain, Dr. Usui was able, using the symbols, to do three healings on himself. And his faith in the sacred healing symbols was confirmed.

Dr. Usui then went into the poor section of Kyoto and began healing people, but he soon found that after the healings many people simply resumed their former lives, their former "sickness." From this and other experiences, he developed two of the key precepts of Reiki: For healing to take place, first there must be an exchange of energy; that is, the healing must have some value to the recipient. Second there must be a change of consciousness; that is, the recipient of the healing must "draw in" the healing energy and be subconsciously willing to be changed by the healing.

When he returned to Tokyo, Usui created a healing system based on the ancient Taoist energy practices widely used at that time. His system, known as *Usui Shiki Ryoho* (Usui Natural Healing System), used acupressure points by placing hands on each chakra to release energy blockages in the recipient. Since *Reiki* is a general word in Japan, used for many kinds of healing and spiritual work, Usui's natural healing method became *Usui Reiki*. In Usui Reiki training, the symbols, the procedure, and the healing energy are transmitted from teacher to student in a secret and sacred attunement process.

The word *Reiki* is made up of two Japanese characters: *rei*, meaning spirit of God, and *ki*, meaning life force. *Rei* also means the essence of All That Is, including everything, living and nonliving, in the universe. It is spiritually directed universal energy. Rei is the transcendental Spirit we call God; it is the field of pure, creative intelligence that brings forth all matter, all existence. It is this Universal Energy that flows through our hands in concentrated form when we use our hands for healing. Ki is the consciousness of the human body, the Life Force Energy. In various cultures, this life force is known as *prana, mana, elan vital,* or *ka*. There must be a free flow of ki to all parts of the body-mind-soul in order for a person to have full health.

Reiki is founded on the natural and ancient law that illness or dis-ease is a matter of being out of balance or out of harmony with ourselves and the Universe. Reiki brings together the God Energy of the Universe and the Life Force of the body, creating a powerful force that flows through the meridians, or energy rivers, into the hands. In a Reiki healing, practitioners pass healing energy to their clients by drawing a series of Japanese and Tibetan symbols over the fully clothed body, accessing the vibratory energy field around them. This electromagnetic field holds all negative thoughts and feelings attached to body, mind, and spirit. Reiki acts as a trigger, setting off an accelerated loosening of the energy, causing negative energy to be forced to the surface and released.

Reiki supports the body's natural ability to heal itself. During healing, we breathe evenly, regularly, naturally. As our breath flows in an easy, relaxed, rhythmic way, so our ki flows in the same way. By balancing the body, Reiki loosens up any areas that are rigid and allows the flow of natural energy through the body, mind, and spirit of the recipient. If we're too cold, it warms us. If we're too warm, it cools us. Reiki restores us to wholeness.

REIKI HEALING AND THE ARCHETYPAL REIKI CARDS

I came to create Archetypal Reiki and the Reiki Healing Cards through my study of Reiki and two other great traditions: the archetypal psychology of Carl Jung and the ancient divination system known as Tarot, using the basic, indigenous context of Japanese Shinto. I have found that the blend of these systems creates a powerful new healing tool for personal and spiritual transformation. Like the Tarot, the Reiki cards contain many layers of meaning. Keep a beginner's mind as you work with them and you'll find new layers of wisdom.

Archetypes are universal patterns of energy, much like our DNA patterns. There are archetypes, or energy forms, for all human qualities and behaviors. For example, the Mona Lisa is an archetype of the enigmatic woman. A particularly puzzling woman in our lives would be the archetype filled in. Another archetype is love. The particular way I love people or animals in my life is the way the pattern is filled in. Archetypes change and develop as we grow and develop. For example, prayer is an archetypal energy form. The particular way that I pray changed as I went from childhood to adulthood.

Archetypes function in the psyche as the facilitator of the union of opposites: positive and negative, dark and light. And it is in the resolution of the tension between opposing forces that we experience growth. Archetypal Reiki helps us to work through and resolve the tension present within ourselves, symbolized by the archetypes found in the Healing Cards and the ways that we handle them. As we do the psychological, emotional, and spiritual work of the cards, we heal our inconsistencies.

There are twenty-eight Archetypal Reiki Cards. Their names come from Reiki tradition, Shinto practices, and general spiritual disciplines. Each card represents an archetype important to our healing work and each has been charged with Reiki energy.

The twenty-eight cards fall naturally into four groups of seven each. Each group is called a cycle, a small path of spiritual growth.

Cycle I: THE DOORWAY OF AWAKENING THROUGH THE SYMBOLS

The way to access power in the Reiki tradition is through the symbol system outlined in Cycle I. Each symbol is a separate mantra (a sacred formula used for invoking the Divinity) representing various forms of enlightenment, and each has its own healing power. Each symbol is complete in and of itself, but working through the cycle as a spiritual exercise, we move from turning on the Light and embracing our dark selves to wholeness of spirit.

Cycle II: WALKING THE PATH TO YOUR TRUTH

Each card in this cycle represents an attribute that is highly desired in spiritual work. Authenticity and emotional discipline are prerequisites to the spiritual values of clear desire and pure intent. By becoming centered in our spirituality and open to Divine revelation, we learn to trust the Universe and transcend our human flaws—at least a major portion of the time. If we work this path in steps, it leads us from dropping the lies in order to find our truth to transcendence in all aspects of our lives.

Cycle III: THROUGH THE GATEWAY TO INITIATION

The cards in Cycle III show us different power spots on this earth and what they represent in spiritual terms. We begin with willingness to enter a spiritual gateway and to perform the necessary ritual of purification in which we drop the "robes of the city" to become aligned with the Reiki Healing Energy. We gain mastery over our ego, our worldly self, and we demonstrate reverence and respect for all things in the Universe. In this way, we get ever closer to the wisdom that we desire. Walking the steps of the third cycle of spiritual development ensures our commitment to the "Shrine of the Soul," in which we contact our personal soul at the end of this leg of our journey.

Cycle IV: FOLLOWING THE CHAKRA PATH TO EMPOWERMENT

The East Indian chakra system correlates closely with the physical endocrine system. Most healing work is done on the seven major chakras running down the center of the body, by laying hands either directly on the body or in the aura slightly above the body. In Archetypal Reiki Card work, these spinning, cone-shaped vortices (centers) of energy are used to evoke different or altered states of consciousness (awareness) through the cards. We begin with the root chakra at the base of the spine, which gives us physical energy. We proceed up the body to creativity and sexuality, at the level of our spleen chakra. From there we become personally empowered through our solar plexus chakra. When we reach the level of the heart chakra, we exchange love with the Universe and with others. Once we know love, we can move into the higher levels of spirituality, open communication with the Divine, gain insight about the purpose of life, and finally, attain oneness with All That Is.

To find the power in the chakras, we meditate upon each chakra card, building one upon the other as we move through this cycle of energy. The chakras form our basic perceptual system, the lens through which we view our world. Balanced chakras result in maximum vitality and health.

Throughout this book you will find suggestions on how to work with the cards. Once you begin to experience the power of Archetypal Reiki, you will undoubtedly come up with your own methods for working with them.

When we draw a card and see the image, we embrace the dark side of that archetype (or of ourselves) as well as the light side. For example, if you draw the Intent and Purpose card, you will be working with the two poles of that archetype. One pole of desire and intent is purity and clarity (pure intent/clear purpose). The opposite pole is ill will and accident or purposelessness. If the card is upright when chosen, you are being shown that you have pure intent but your head is in the clouds and you need grounding. If the card is reversed, you will want to work on resolving feelings of ill will. As we fully enter each archetype and its energy, we integrate both extremes into our psyche; we become balanced; we become whole.

It is important to remember that healing is an ongoing process. In the material world, we think of healing as a cure for the physical body, that disease originates in the physical body and the material world. In this view, a cure would mean a restoration of the physical body to its original health. In the metaphysical world, the cause for all disease, dis-comfort, and illness is spiritual, a disharmony, a splittingoff of our spiritual nature into fragmented pieces. A restoration to oneness, to holy health, does not necessarily mean physical health, though it certainly can occur.

We must remember the concept of the hologram: One card or any number of cards pulled "at random" will provide information about the whole, because everything is interconnected and interdependent.

When you work with the Archetypal Reiki Cards, notice your hands as they move toward or away from a particular card or cards. Our hand chakras are vital centers of psychic energy and spontaneous expressions of our unconscious mind. Notice sensations of temperature, a magnetic pulling or drawing of the hand to a particular card, tingling or little electric shocks, feelings of pins and needles or bursting of little bubbles on your skin. As you work with Archetypal Reiki you may even feel a deep, rhythmic pulsation of the ki within or experience deep insights into your own or someone else's condition or situation. When you do, you'll know you are in touch with the creative energy of the universe.

ONE Getting Started

When doing any healing work it is important to slow down to hear the voice of intuition. Speed up and the voice of ego echoes in our ears. Healing work also requires that we create some sacred space. It can be a special room, a corner of a room, or a favorite spot outdoors in nature. It's up to you. Think of creating some sacred space inside yourself as well.

CREATING SACRED SPACE

DEDICATE THE SPACE. Dedication of space means that we reverently declare our intention to set it apart from other space and consecrate it for this particular work. One simple way to dedicate space is to state aloud, "I, [your name], dedicate myself and this space to the work that needs to be done."

SET ASIDE TIME. Interruptions break the energy cycle. Make sure to have quiet, uninterrupted time for your work with the Reiki Cards—anywhere from five minutes to three hours. It's up to you.

BUILD AN ALTAR. An altar is an important tool for focusing and grounding. It can be as simple as a table; a large, flat rock; or a place on the ground. Place items on the altar that have unique meaning or value to you. They can be items you've collected or that have been given to you by someone special. Arrange them in an order that is pleasing to you. Any of the following (and many others) are appropriate altar items: candles, pictures, statues, stones, feathers, cards, essential oils, a favorite pendulum, and any reading or writing material you desire.

PERFORM A RITUAL. Rituals solidify a spiritual discipline. A prayer can be a ritual or part of a ritual. Rituals are transitional devices that allow the conscious mind to let go and the unconscious mind to take over. They can be as simple as lighting a candle or ringing a small gong. Their purpose is to call your attention to what you intend to do here and to keep your mind focused on the spiritual work at hand.

MAKE AN INVOCATION. Say a prayer or invocation at the beginning of your session. Use the words, preferably spoken aloud, to call forth your God, spirit guides, or any other spiritual aids you need.

SET AN INTENTION. Set your intention, preferably aloud, by asking for what you desire. Ask in the present tense, as if it has already happened. For example, "I intend to have abundance in my life. There is enough [time] to do all I want to do. There is enough [love] to be all I desire to be."

CHOOSE YOUR TOOLS. Before you enter your sacred space, choose the spiritual tool or tools you will need for your intention and desire. A spiritual tool can be as simple as a single prayer. It can be a card reading, a spiritual writing or reading, or anything that helps you communicate with the Divine.

CLOSE your healing session with a prayer of gratitude for all you've been given.

BLESSING THE CARDS

The first time you use a new deck of cards or any other spiritual tool, take the time to dedicate or bless it so that it will have your energy on it and that of the spirits you have around you. Take your unopened deck and place it on your altar. Say a special prayer of blessing, such as: "Dear God, Dear Spirit Guides, I dedicate myself and these cards to Your work. I ask your blessings and your help as I do the work that is before me to do. Stay with me always and allow only positive energy to be circulated around these cards. Amen. So be it. It is done."

Then open the cards and begin by handling them one by one so, individual energy mingles with that of the cards. As this is done, think only positive thoughts and set your intention to be a force for "good."

SHUFFLING THE DECK

Unless the particular method you're using states otherwise, shuffle the Reiki Healing Cards in any way that feels intuitively right. Turn half the cards upside down so that when the cards are laid out, some will be upright and others will be reversed. This deliberate act of being willing to look at the other side of an archetype, a quality or principle, is a very important act of faith. Shuffle the cards again.

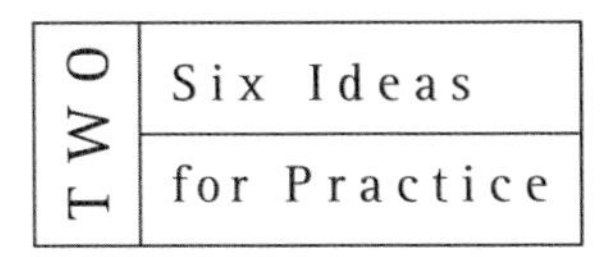

TWO Six Ideas for Practice

The Archetypal Reiki Cards may be used in an infinite number of ways. In this chapter you will find six ideas for practice: daily readings; intuitive readings; readings involving going to your very center, your tantien; readings that call upon your spirit guides; readings as oracle; and readings as a meditative tool. Try each of these practices and stick with the ones that work best for you. Of course, you can create your own methods, too. The sky's the limit.

ONE: DAILY PRACTICE

Archetypal Reiki Cards can be used as a daily practice in themselves or they can be combined with other practices. Some people "practice" in the morning, some in the evening. Whatever works best for you. What is important is that you do it every day. In this way, you commit to the development of your spiritual practice.

> We have to go beyond our practices. It isn't only the practice . . . that makes us sweet and clear . . . it is our willingness to experiment, to go to God beyond old conditioning, beyond old anything, beyond old seconds just passed . . . It's the heart that does the practice that counts.
>
> —Stephen Levine

FOLLOW THE GENERAL INSTRUCTIONS for "Getting Started" (page 15).

FAN OUT THE DECK, facedown, and choose one card at random.

LAY THE CARD in front of you, facedown, and say a short prayer of invocation.

ASK YOUR GUIDES and teachers to be with you and to guide your thinking and feeling on a particular issue, or just to provide a focus for the day. You may say, as I often do, "Light my way and direct my feet on my path of truth."

MEDITATE on the card. Turn the card over and look at it without thinking. Bring your attention down from your head through your body into that stillpoint around your belly, your tantien. From that stillpoint, meditate on the card for as long as you like—a few moments or half an hour—it's up to you.

JOURNAL your impressions of the card and the answer the card has shown you.

READ THE TEACHINGS in the second half of this book. Notice which words "jump out at you," which words seem to speak to your deepest essence. Go beyond the concrete, literal meaning of the words—to the spirit of the words and to the space between the words where Spirit moves. If you wish to go deeper, do the suggested meditation.

JOURNAL AGAIN. You will find a clear answer. If an answer does not appear clearly, either it is not time to deal with that particular issue or situation or you need to do more internal work on it.

TWO: INTUITIVE READINGS

Intuition is a powerful ally in Archetypal Reiki work; it draws us to the particular work we need to do and offers us invaluable guidance in that work.

Intuition is our inner knowing system. It comes to us from a soft, gentle voice deep within us and always operates in our own best interests, though intuitive messages may challenge and divert us from a path we thought we needed to follow. Intuitive information is never misleading. If we are to participate consciously in the evolution of our souls, we need to trust that our intuition is a form of spiritual communication from our deepest essence. If we trust our intuition, it will guide us to the right spiritual tool at the right time. But we must do the "legwork" on a daily basis.

USING INTUITION IN ARCHETYPAL REIKI CARD WORK

When you want to hear the voice of intuition through the Reiki Healing Cards,

FOLLOW THE GENERAL INSTRUCTIONS for "Getting Started" (page 15).

SHUFFLE THE FULL DECK. Frame your question carefully and specifically. "My Dear Intuition: Tell me what to do about ___" or "What is the purpose of ___ in my life today?" Or, for a more general answer, you might ask: "What does my intuition have to say to me today?"

DRAW TWO CARDS. Lay them facedown, first one to the left, second one to the right. The card on the left will be a general answer, while the card on the right will be more specific.

MEDITATE. Journal. Read the teachings. Journal again. Your answer will be clear. If more clarity is needed, it is well to ask for further clarification. A simple "I need clarification on this issue, please."

BE SURE TO THANK the voice of your intuition for appearing to you today.

THREE: USING ARCHETYPAL REIKI AND THE TANTIEN

The tantien (don-d-en) is a physical center in the body, right above the pelvic bone and about four inches below the navel. It is known by several names: stillpoint, one point, center, hara. Think of the physical sacrum or lower back, right below the five vertebrae. This is the tantien.

This point has no definable size or position, although we can visualize it in certain ways. Its position shifts farther down whenever the upper body leans forward or bends back, and it is capable of infinite expansion or contraction. It is like the lowest point in a strong whirlpool. The tantien acts like a miniature star, radiating ki out or funneling it in from all directions. By focusing on this point we release all stress from the body and mind. The body becomes light and buoyant, free from unnecessary tension or restriction. Allow the weight of every part of the body to settle naturally at its lowest point. Gravity naturally seeks the weight of any object's underside without any help from us. Life energy is in the belly, not the heart or head. Before doing the following exercise, draw three cards from the full deck. Place them in front of you faceup and look at them carefully. Ask to feel the energy of your tantien and to hear the message it sends. Then do the following exercise:

THE EXERCISE can be done in a sitting or a standing position. Keep the spine straight and the legs firm (or feet flat on the floor) while breathing deeply from the belly.

MAKE AN INVERTED TRIANGLE with your hands and place it just above your pelvic line, with index fingers together at the bottom and thumbs touching at the top. This is the center point or tantien. From this point the breath of ki flows, and in this center ki can be stored or moved around the body and the environment.

CLOSE YOUR EYES and breathe slowly and deeply. Breathe into your abdomen. Visualize the tantien. Allow your breath to enter your body in a golden flow through your tantien. Once you have taken in a full breath, hold it for a moment and release the breath while visualizing the golden flow.

Silently AFFIRM with feeling: "I am completely still and at peace. I breathe through my tantien and rest within the heart of the Universe."

WHEN YOU FEEL FINISHED, look at the three cards again; take out your Archetypal Reiki journal and write about your experience.

FOUR: WORKING WITH SPIRIT GUIDES

It is said in the Reiki tradition that a group of people who lived in Tibet before Buddhism, at the time of the Bon religion, were greatly evolved spiritually and saw into the future. They anticipated our need and created an energy pattern that would be used to assist us in this time. This energy pattern was Dr. Usui's Reiki. An understanding of the spirit world is vital to Reiki. When we are attuned to Reiki energy, the entire troop of Reiki guides, teachers, and Reiki masters are available to us. We call upon them each and every time we do any kind of Reiki healing work. They never let us down nor will they abandon us. There may also be one or two special Reiki guides who are specific to an individual, our own internal Reiki healers, and they will appear to help us in this sacred work.

Here's a good method for invoking your spirit guides in your work with the Archetypal Reiki Cards:

FOLLOW THE INSTRUCTIONS for getting started (page 15).

INVOKE your spirit guides and image them.

TO SEE which one you need for your current issue, shuffle the cards and select five, laying them out in the following pattern:

Place the first card facedown on the table.

Place the second card in a new row, facedown on your left.

Place the third card facedown in the middle of the row.

Place the fourth card facedown on your right of the row.

Place the fifth card in a new, bottom row, facedown.

The first card is the issue at hand. The second is the spirit guide of the past, the one whose help you have needed on this issue in the recent past. The third card is the spirit guide of the present, the one who is guiding you on this issue now. The fourth card is the spirit guide of the future, the one who will be coming into your life in the near future to help with this issue. The fifth card is the lesson to be learned from this issue.

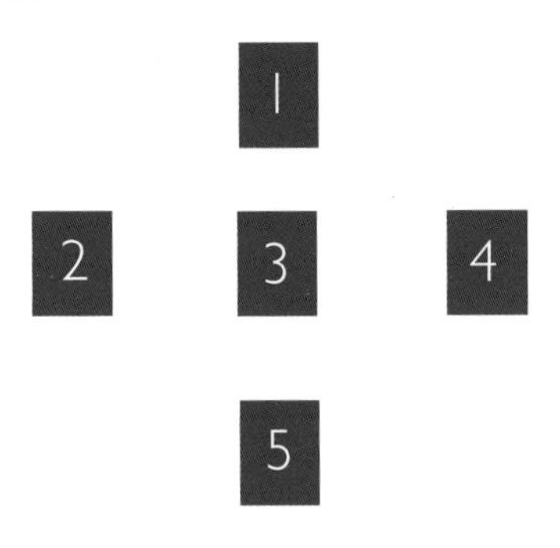

WHEN YOU HAVE FINISHED THIS READING, thank your spirit guides and be sure to refer to the ones helping you on this issue for at least the next week.

FIVE: WORKING WITH ORACLES: SPIRIT GUIDES WITH A TWIST

Oracles are another kind of spirit guide. Evidence suggests that people have been consulting oracles throughout human history. They are messengers of God and can be used for guidance. An oracle will always lead you to your own highest purpose and will never interfere with anyone else's path.

Oracles usually come to us in the form of signs or symbols. The Oracle of Delphi is the most well known oracle, but numerology, astrology, the I Ching, Runes, Angel Cards, and Archetypal Reiki are all forms of oracles. Palm readings, power places, Tarot cards, and almost anything found in nature has been consulted for oracular wisdom.

An oracular message can be given through our own heart, mind, or intuition.

If the message feels right, if it resonates with your deepest essence, then chances are you can trust it. As always, we must be very careful when consulting oracles or when interpreting various messages that we don't take a messianic stance. Humility is at the heart of any spiritual practice.

You may use any of the methods or layouts to hear the oracle speak, but there are several specific things we can do to strengthen your relationship with oracular knowing:

Remember that God is the Source. The oracle is the mediator.

Be patient with respect to discovering oracles.

Approach your practice with reverence and humility.

Maintain a structured ritual setting for divination.

State your sacred intention, aloud when possible.

Do not ask the same question two times in a row, though you may ask for clarification. To keep asking the same question over and over shows lack of faith.

Do not become tied to the messages of the oracle.

Always check your own inner knowing.

End with a prayer of gratitude for the help received.

SIX: USING THE CARDS AS A MEDITATIVE TOOL

Meditation is the foundation of all spiritual discipline. It is also an extremely beneficial physical and emotional practice. In meditation we try to get past the control of the conscious mind, of our ego. We allow ourselves to relax and the fragmented parts of us to coalesce and become whole. Meditation is not just expanded knowing but expanded being, and there are as many meditation techniques as there are spiritual teachers. It connects us with our deepest Self and with our Source. Meditation calms and focuses our lives and connects us to God and to others. Let's look at some principles of meditation as it is used in deepening our Archetypal Reiki work.

The *subconscious mind* does not know the difference between "real" and "imagined" information. In meditation, if you want change, you must reach your subconscious (nonthinking) mind.

Use all your *senses and all colors* to make the meditations vivid and real.

Determine your *primary mode* of accessing information. We use all the modalities, but there is usually one that is strongest for each of us.

If you process information visually (see pictures), use the word *See*.

If you are more kinesthetic (feeling your body sensations in space), say "Feel."

If you are auditory (tending to hear instructions), say "Hear."

If you are a knower (just "knowing" something deep inside), say "Know."

If your primary mode is imagination (picture, think, intuit, infer), say "Imagine."

Use a *relaxation induction* to gain entry into your own essential core being. One relaxation induction is Relax your body. Relax your mind. Take three deep breaths, in and out, rhythmically, naturally, and easily. Let go of time. You have all the time you need.

DO NOT THINK. Only be still. When thoughts come into your mind, allow them to flow gently past your awareness. And breathe.

GO INTO A PLACE deep within the center of yourself. This is a quiet place, a safe place, a holy space. It is deep within the center of you. Be there now. Breathe.

From that space see, feel, know, imagine . . . (use your primary modality).

AFTER A TIME, this process can be shortened: Put yourself in the quiet, safe, sacred space that has become familiar to you. Be there now. Breathe fully and deeply. With practice, you can simply breathe yourself into a sacred space. Affirm the presence of your Higher Self and your spirit guides. Be there now. Breathe into that space.

When using Archetypal Reiki Cards as a meditation, draw one card and meditate on it either with a specific question in mind or for general guidance. The card can give you a "progress report."

Separate the card you drew from the rest of the deck and meditate on it daily for a week. Think about the principles it symbolizes during this time, and every day, deepen your meditation and your application (how these principles concretely apply to your life).

Archetypal Reiki Cards are versatile and flexible. Using the cards daily will add to any spiritual practice you have created. Spiritual work is mysterious, but we know that our intuition must be developed in order to access our deeper selves. We view the tantien as a spiritual center within us that, with practice, can be reached. The cards may be used as a vehicle for contacting our spirit guides and as oracular guidance on a daily, weekly, or monthly basis. As a meditative tool, Archetypal Reiki Cards produce astonishing results. Other methods will be given, but in the basic practice, we use all of the ways we have just discussed.

THREE

Ten Layouts

In this section, we will look at ten layouts using the Reiki Healing Cards. Each layout, created for variety and interest in Archetypal Reiki Card work, has a specific purpose, such as when we need to change direction or to find more balance, or when we reach a plateau in creative work. Cards from a well-shuffled deck are laid out on a table in a prescribed pattern, which is then interpreted. These patterns are similar to the archetypes in that they are empty forms that we fill in, according to desire and intent.

GENERAL TIPS ON USING THE LAYOUTS

BEFORE YOU DO A CARD LAYOUT, create your sacred space and get your Reiki Healing Journal.

SHUFFLE THE CARDS in any manner you desire. In the layouts there are no reversals, so it is important that you arrange all the cards in the upright position before shuffling or turn them right-side up if they appear reversed.

AFTER SHUFFLING, put the deck on the table facedown and spread it out, creating a "fan" effect.

PASS YOUR HAND OVER EACH CARD, stopping over any card that calls to you. Your hand may tingle, grow warm, get cooler, or you may just get "a feeling" or "a hunch." This is the card your unconscious mind has chosen. This is the card to use in the layout. You may wish to draw from the top of the deck, the bottom, or the middle. Follow your intuition in this matter. Remember that personal intent and desire is the foundation of all spiritual work.

Since the position of the card in a layout is all-important, be sure to lay out the cards in the sequence in which they are chosen.

STEPPING ACROSS THE THRESHOLD

This layout helps us step across the threshold of the day to explore what the day holds for us. The card you draw will show you the treasure of today and where you can begin to make the day's potential a reality.

DRAW A CARD from the shuffled, fanned-out deck or from the top of the shuffled deck.

TURN THE CARD over slowly and process the meaning of the card for you and your life. After recording your impressions in your journal, turn to the card section of the book for the teachings.

DATE AND JOURNAL your final responses and your "answers."

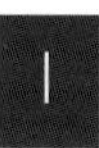

LIGHT AND DARK, OPPOSING ENERGIES

From the newly shuffled deck, draw two cards as you realize two different energies today. Lay them out in opposition to one another. The cards you choose will operate in one of the following ways:

To show you your Golden Shadow, or positive potential, and your Dark Shadow, your negative potential.
To show you two choices or two alternatives.
To show you your conflict.
To show you the two opposing energies you must unite.

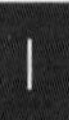

2

A DYNAMIC PROCESS

From the newly shuffled deck, draw three cards as you realize that your spirituality is a dynamic process. Lay the cards out in a triangle in the order in which they were selected. The cards will show one or more of the following things:

1. The beginning, middle, and end of your current project.
2. The past, present, and future.
3. Any triangle or trinity or triune that is operating in your life today.

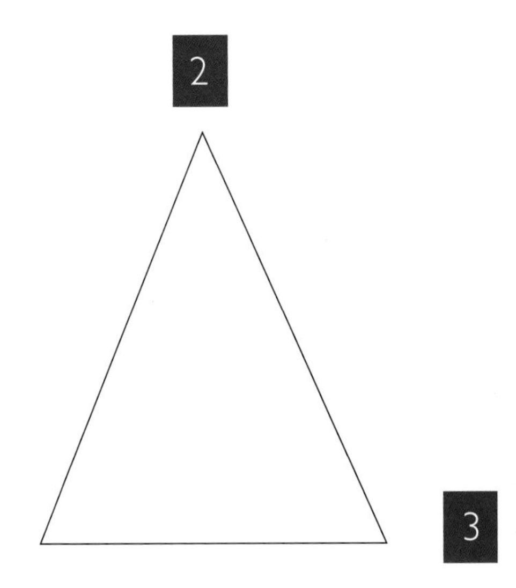

A PLATEAU

From the newly shuffled deck, draw four cards as you realize you have come to a natural plateau in your strivings. Lay the cards out in the form of a square. The cards will point out a pattern in the following order:

1. What is coming to completion.
2. What the boundaries of the situation are.
3. Your inner organization on the issue at hand.
4. How you can stabilize the changes in your life.

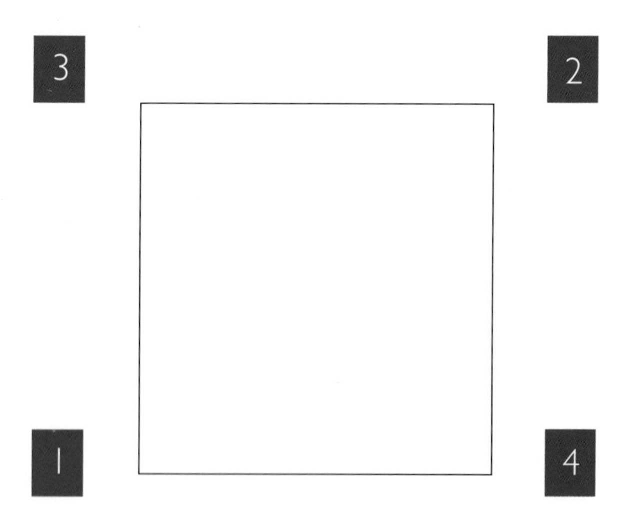

CHANGING DIRECTION

From the newly shuffled deck, draw five cards as you come to an opportunity to actively change direction in your life. Lay out the cards in the shape of a five-pointed star. You will see:

1. What is grounding you and what you are reaching for.
2. Where to take action.
3. What your inner struggle is about.
4. How to make your own personal vision a reality in the outer world.
5. What tests you will be facing in your current life situation.

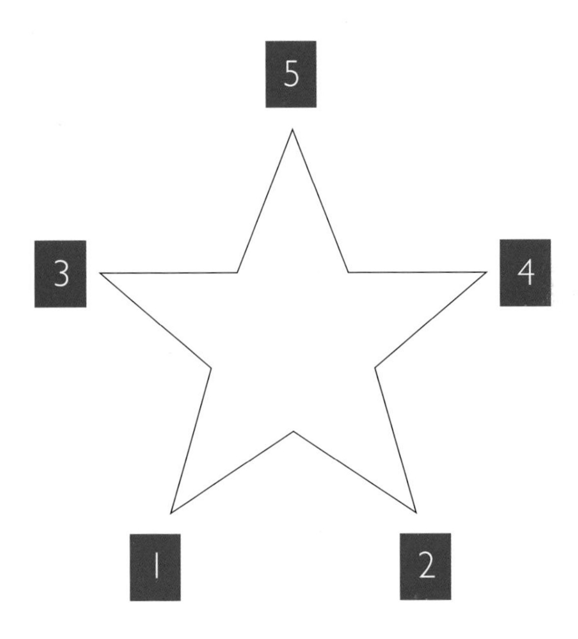

A PAUSE IN CREATIVE WORK

From the newly shuffled deck, draw six cards as you recognize that you have come to a pause that follows the completion of a phase of your creative work (whether it's a creative project, creating a child, or creating a day). Lay out the cards in the form of yin-yang (see illustration) and they will tell you:

1. The opposing forces within your heart that you have united.
2. Where you are to look for guidance.
3. What is balanced in your life.
4. In what ways your spirituality is deepening.
5. What needs integration in your life or within yourself.
6. Where to go from here.

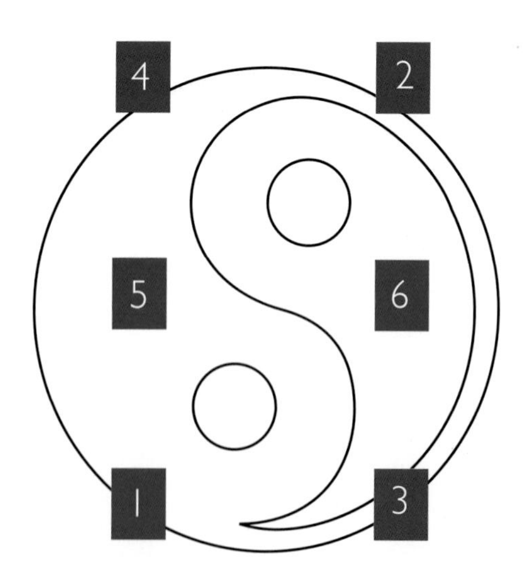

A RESOLUTION AND NEW TESTS

From the newly shuffled deck, draw seven cards as you recognize that something has been resolved. Lay out the cards in a rainbow shape (see illustration) and they will tell you:

1. What your current tests are.
2. What your current obstacles are.
3. Where you will have an increase in energy, ideas, or insight.
4. In what ways you will find movement in your current situation.
5. Who your teacher is in this situation.
6. How you can develop your ideas.
7. What your Higher Self advises about the situation.

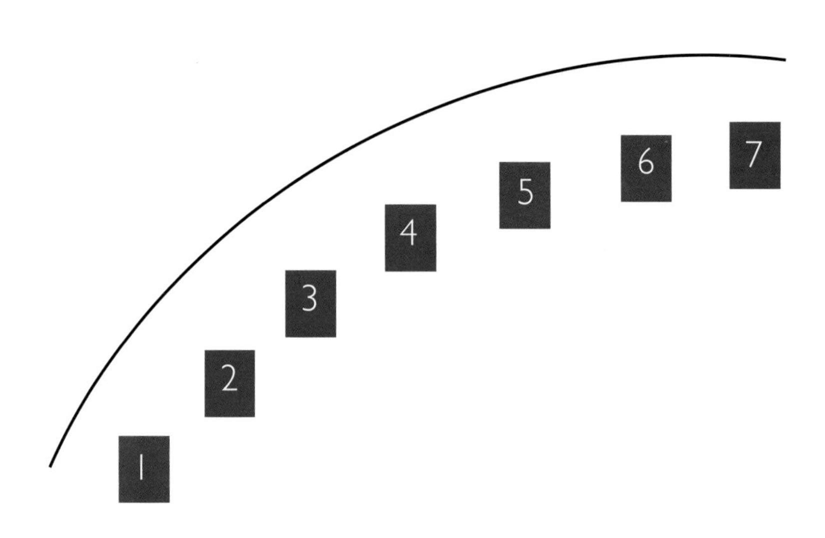

BALANCE

From the newly shuffled deck, draw eight cards as you realize that your life is fairly well balanced and harmonized at this point—or the opposite, that you are greatly in need of balance and harmony. Lay out the cards in the form of the infinity sign and they will show you:

1. What has been stabilized.
2. What is resurrecting or coming back into your life situation or yourself.
3. What comes before the next significant change in your life or in yourself.
4. One choice you face immediately.
5. An opposing choice or another alternative.
6. The resolution of the two.
7. What needs to be reevaluated and prioritized.
8. The next step before rebirth.

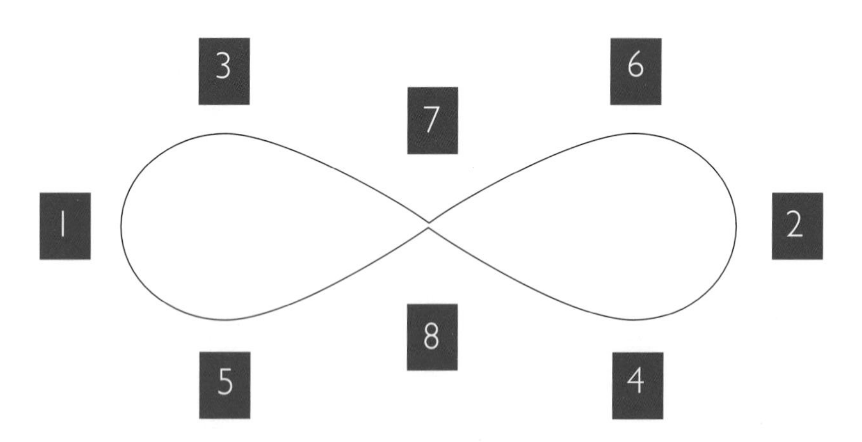

SPIRIT GUIDES

From the newly shuffled deck, draw nine cards as you feel the presence of benevolent spiritual beings in your life. Lay out the cards in the shape of three interconnecting circles and they will tell you:

1. The issue at hand.
2. Your conscious desire.
3. Your unconscious desire.
4. What your inner fulfillment is all about.
5. What your inner wisdom says.
6. Where you have been successful.
7. What is synthesized in your life situation or in yourself right now.
8. What needs to be integrated before the new birth.
9. Who is helping you at this time of your life.

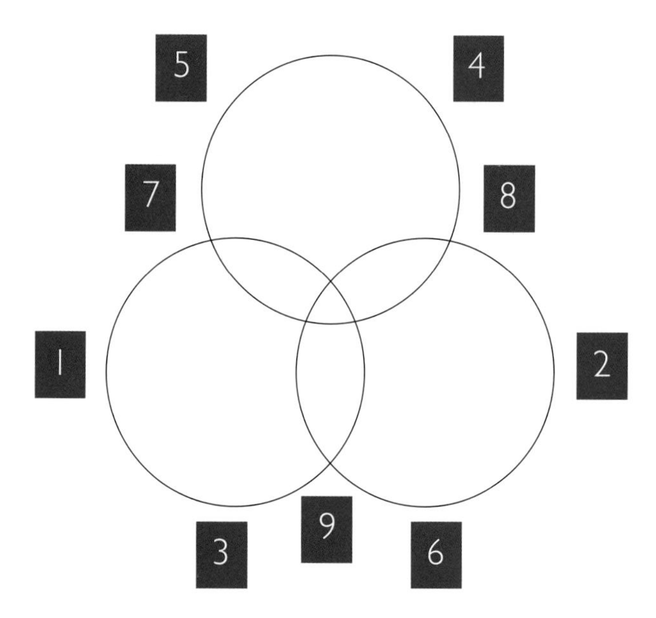

UNITY

From the newly shuffled deck, draw ten cards as you feel a return to unity. Lay them out in the form of two hands side by side and they will tell you:

1. When this cycle began.
2. The purpose of this cycle.
3. What is culminating now.
4. What it is you want.
5. What is holding you back.
6. The seeds of the beginning are in the ending. This card shows the ending.
7. What it is that you cannot release.
8. What it is that you rebel against.
9. There is a group of elders or wise people advising or supporting you. This card shows who they are.
10. How you can begin the next cycle of growth.

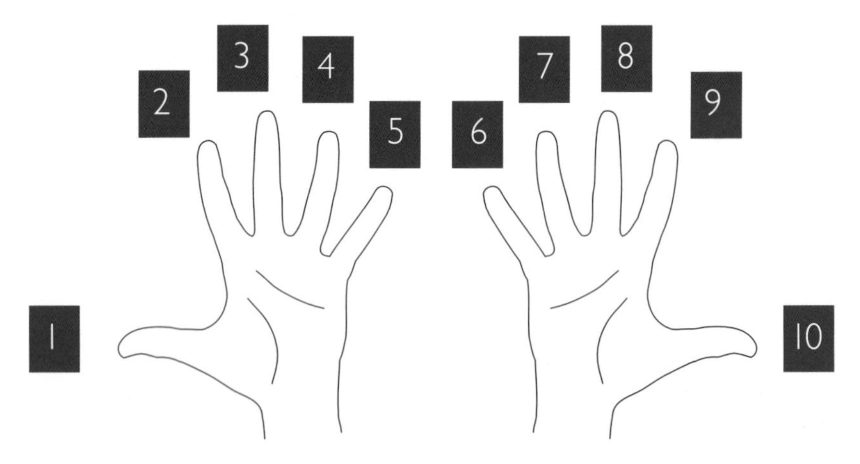

We use layouts for whatever purpose we desire. For an overview of your spiritual path, to see where you've been and where you're going, turn to "Chapter Four, Archetypal Reiki Pathwork."

FOUR Archetypal Reiki Pathwork

Archetypal Reiki Pathwork is a map of your archetypal spiritual evolution. The goal of this work is to integrate different parts of you, to unify and embrace the opposite energy forces within you, and to accept the wholeness that is you: mind, body, heart, and soul.

Pathwork will help you to trace your path by following the healing archetype as it appeared in your life in the past. The healing archetype can appear in any concrete form: as synchronicities leading you in a particular way toward your healing; as a health crisis experienced by you or a loved one; as choosing to do healing work such as becoming a doctor, a teacher, a nurse, a mother, a lawyer, or any other kind of helping work; as a near-death experience. These experiences represent the lessons we are to learn in life, as each one requires a healing and a wholing.

From reflection on the past, you can find new direction, still following the healing archetype as it shows itself to you now, in your current life. If you desire, the cards can also lead you toward a future path.

Using either the entire deck or the split deck in the Wheel method gives you an overall view of your personal soul (Self) in relation to the Universal Energy (Spirit). When you have viewed all twenty-eight cards and journaled, the map will emerge. Using the Story method shows you how your specific healing path originated, and if you write your vision metaphorically (a metaphor is an image that carries a specific meaning, such as "the evening of life"), the map will emerge.

In Archetypal Reiki Pathwork, as in the other methods described in this book, the cards that appear frequently over time are those that need your attention. So Archetypal Reiki Pathwork should be done at turning points in your life, when you know something important is happening but you can't quite put your finger on what it is.

All the cards should face the same way. There are no reversals in pathwork. In these sessions, you can work with the entire deck or with a split deck.

BEGIN EACH PATHWORK SESSION WITH THE FOLLOWING RITUAL

DO AN INVOCATION, asking your spirit guides to help you.

DEDICATE yourself to your spiritual path.

APPRECIATE all you've been given.

OFFER THIS PRAYER: "In my center there is a stillness. The fragmented pieces of my life surround me."

WORKING WITH THE ENTIRE DECK

Whether we use the entire deck or the split deck, we walk the path according to the choices of our unconscious mind.

Arrange the cards in numerical order. Draw one card at each sitting. In the first session, draw the first card, the Doorway. Meditate on how this archetype applies to your life and journal your results. In the second session, draw the second card, Release Bound-Up Energy. Again, meditate on how this archetype applies to your life and journal your results. Proceed through each card, and when all have been completed, a map of your spiritual evolution will be clear.

Both sides of the archetype are valuable to spiritual evolution. Do not judge or ignore either extreme. Know only that the extreme of a quality, principle, or characteristic is what is harmful; while a relative balance or harmony is what is helpful.

WORKING WITH A SPLIT DECK

When we choose to work with a split deck, we have two options:

THE WHEEL: A METHOD FOR WORKING WITH THE CYCLES OF HEALING

In cycle work, each of the four categories is used as a separate path, cycle, or phase of the work. In this case, the cards are separated into four separate piles and worked with one cycle at a time, beginning with Cycle I and ending with Cycle IV.

Lay out the seven cards of Cycle I in the shape of an imaginary wheel, in a mirror fashion (see illustration). In a meditative state, move around the wheel one card at a time. Begin with the first card.

LOOK AT THE IMAGE of the archetype, Cho Ku Rei, the Doorway of Light, and meditate silently on this picture while repeating the name of the archetype.

JOURNAL your impressions in words or short phrases.

READ the teachings for this card. Take note of both polarities of the archetype.

NOTE where you are on the continuum.

WRITE one paragraph about how this archetype applies to your life.

JOURNAL any insights or messages you receive from this reading.

Do the same for each card in succession until Cycle I has been completed. When you are done, summarize in your journal what it means to you in one or two sentences. Proceed to the other cycles until you have completed them all. When you have finished all four cycles, reread your journal summaries. You will see the map. You will see the strengths, weaknesses, and the gaps of your spiritual journey.

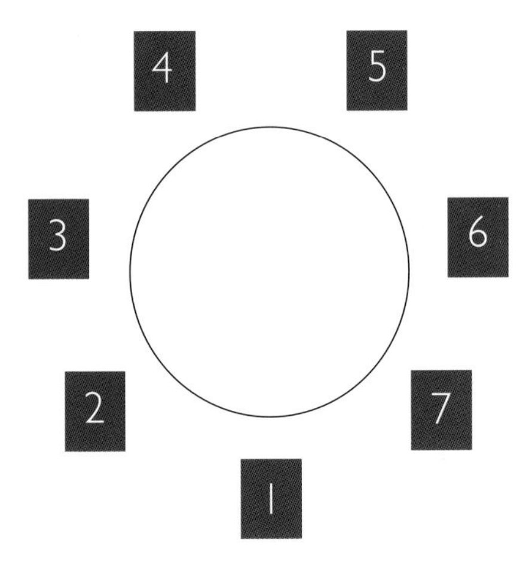

TELLING YOUR STORY METHOD

To work with the Story method; BEGIN BY SHUFFLING the entire deck and drawing a total of three cards. There are no reversals in pathwork, so be sure all the cards are facing in the same direction.

PLACE THE CARDS faceup from left to right on the table. The three cards tell a story. The first one stands for the past, the second one represents the present, and the third one symbolizes the future.

READ the three cards and the parts of the book relating to those cards, look beneath the surface, allow the cards to tell your story and think about three questions:

When did the healing archetype first enter my life? (past)

What does my healing path look like now? (present)

Where will my path lead? (future)

ENVISION your healing path metaphorically, using all of your senses. Metaphors for the path can be landscape, vehicles, a walk through a city, a shamanic journey. Briefly describe this vision in your journal.

The first six methods in this section form the basic practice of the Archetypal Reiki Cards. Layouts and pathwork have been included for special needs. Now that we are familiar and comfortable with the various applications of the Reiki Healing Cards, we turn to the teachings for each card.

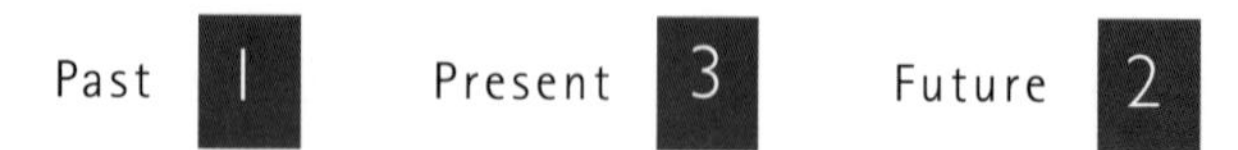

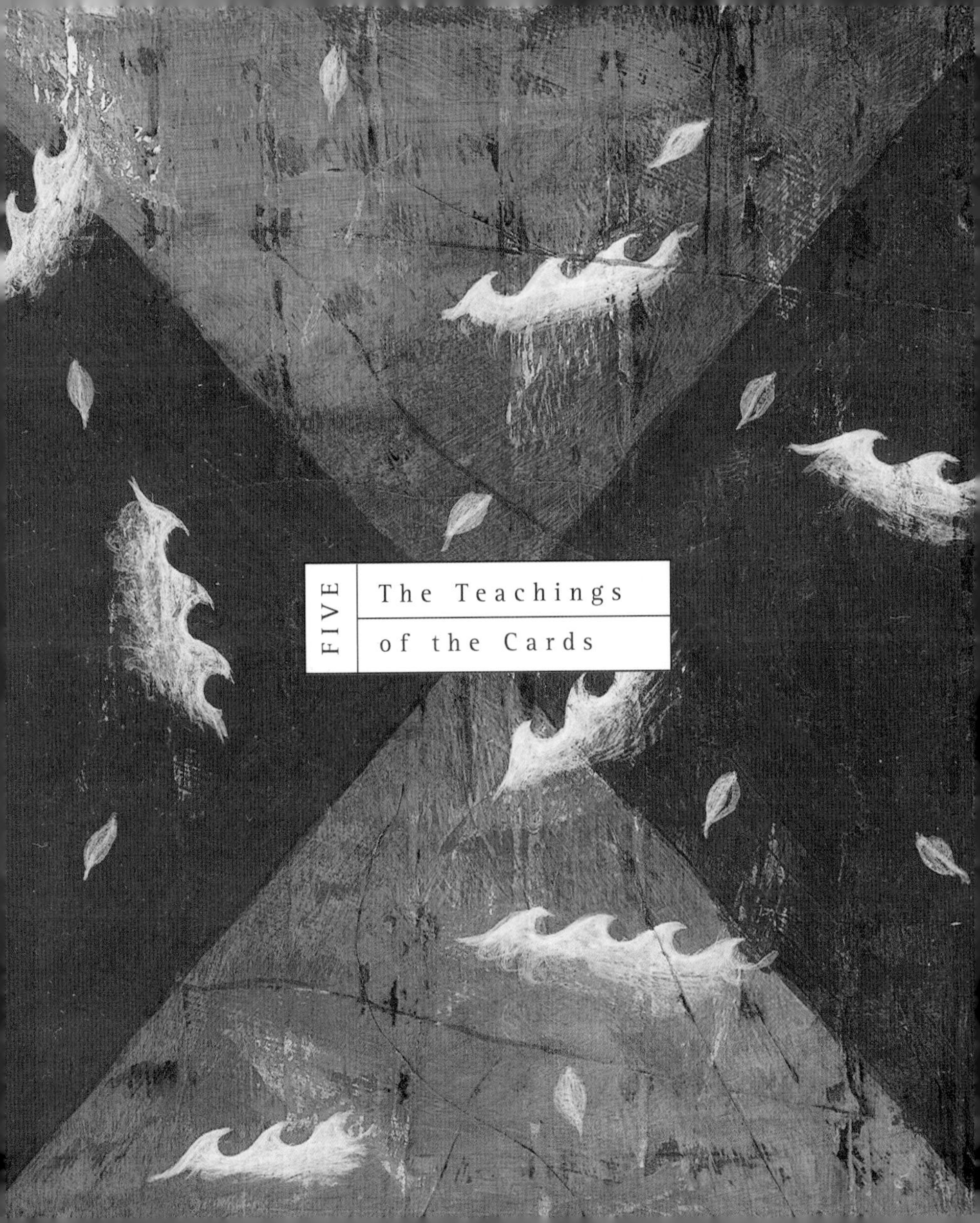

FIVE The Teachings of the Cards

The rest of this book presents the teachings of the cards. For each card, these include an explanation of the archetype, an interpretation of the card when you draw it in a reading, a reflection or exercise, a verbal affirmation, and a meditation that deepens the card experience.

There is no beginning relaxation technique given in the meditations. Before doing the meditations, then, refer to page 22, "Using the Cards as a Meditative Tool." This provides the information needed for successful deepening practice.

I. CHO KU REI: THE DOORWAY OF LIGHT

Be receptive to the gifts you receive from SpiritGod. Stay in the light and notice the shadows dancing on your walls.

Cho Ku Rei (pronounced cho-koo-ray) is one of the four original symbols given to Reiki's founder, Dr. Usui, during his mystical awakening. It is a bridging symbol, the symbol most used for healing in the physical realm, which would include the workplace, money, and safety needs as well as the physical body. In many spiritual traditions, the body is largely ignored; in the Archetypal Reiki system, we begin with the body symbol. Cho Ku Rei is the doorway to the spirit world, which begins with the physical body.

I suggest that you begin your work with this card with a prayer or invocation that speaks to your body as the entryway of healing. One prayer form might be as follows: "As I begin this path of healing, I ask that the work begin with my body. A healing occurs at every level of my physical being. So be it. Thank You."

The polarities within this archetype are light and darkness. If we try to live "in the light" all the time, trying to be too good, too perfect, too spiritual, we tend to ignore our physical life. We deny our human heritage. Our eyes burn out if we stare too long at the sun. Our skins burn up if we stay too long in the sun. Sleep is refreshing. In our sleep, it is dark.

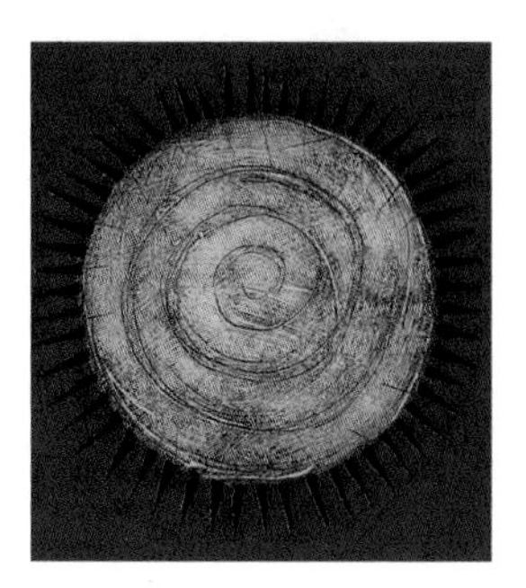

Darkness exists as a shadow of light. If we did not have darkness, we would not know light. When we see the shadows on the wall, we see our human nature. We see our flaws. We see that we are material beings as well as spiritual ones. When we accept and love both our light and our darkness, we are in balance.

WHEN YOU DRAW THIS CARD be receptive to the gifts you receive from SpiritGod.

If the card is UPRIGHT, you take good care of your material well-being. You are asked to move through your physical body into the light of your soul and attend to your spiritual needs.

If the card is REVERSED, your body, financial affairs, your home, or your car need attention. Something may be wrong and you are "in the dark" (unknowing) about it. Embracing the dark means being willing to look at your dark side and acknowledge the messages from your unconscious.

REFLECT on how you might improve the health and well-being of your physical body—or your job, your home, your physical life—so that it truly reflects your ongoing spiritual development.

WRITE down three goals that would improve your physical life and lead you onward spiritually.

AFFIRM with feeling: "Today I honor my physical body, my home, my work. As I care for my physical life, so do I care for my Soul."

CHO KU REI MEDITATION

The meditation for Card No. 1 is a manifestation meditation. *Manifestation* means to bring into the physical world that which begins in the spirit world, and it occurs through intention and desire. It creates a spiritual blueprint, which in turn creates a form in the physical world.

- Declare your wish.
- Visualize, feel, know, or imagine your wish with you in it. Visualize in color and action, with as much detail as you can.
- Place the earth behind it and you on the earth, also in color and detail.
- Position a golden diagonal or spiral grid over the picture running from sky to earth, like a rainbow arch.
- In your mind's eye, draw a doorway, representing Cho Ku Rei, over the whole picture.
- Hold the image for as long as you can.
- Let it go.
- Do not monitor the progress of this goal. But let go of the outcome and . . .
- Surrender it to God's care.
- Be careful what you ask for, you might get it!

2. SEI HEI KI: RELEASE BOUND-UP ENERGY

Let go. Holding tight to something causes blocks in our energy system. Release your hold and let go of control in order to trust the Universe.

Sei Hei Ki (pronounced say-hay-key) is one of the four original Reiki symbols given to Dr. Usui. It involves the release of negative or tension-producing emotions or thoughts. In the Archetypal Reiki system, we use Sei Hei Ki to release emotional debris and negative, outworn mental thought forms.

The word *Sei Hei Ki* is used for emotional, mental, or spiritual protection and purification. If you feel or sense that some negative or unwanted energy is operating in your life, you may use this as a mantra to release that entity or the sense of it.

The polarities within this archetype are detachment and enmeshment. To detach means to set free from emotional confinement, restraint, or bondage. When we detach from an idea, a thought, a feeling, or a person, we release our emotional claim on it. If we detach too much, we become cold and unfeeling. If we detach too soon, we have not given the situation a chance to change. If we detach too late, we become too invested in the situation.

Attachment is a part of our human nature. We want to be close to others. But too much attachment will result in suffocating or smothering. We become enmeshed or embroiled in another person's business, often to the detriment of our own. Too much attachment to an idea or thought will result in overkill and the idea may become useless to us. Too much attachment to our own feelings will result in codependency, a condition that is harmful to our own growth and that of others.

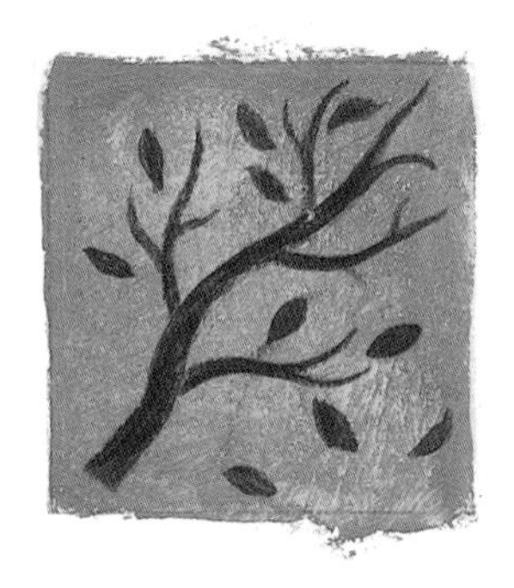

WHEN YOU DRAW THIS CARD you are being asked to examine where in your body you feel tightness, tension. Look at where you are holding on to something that needs to be released.

If the card is UPRIGHT, you work well with the concept of detachment. You must watch that you do not detach too much or too quickly from others. Too much detachment results in emotional irresponsibility.

If the card is REVERSED, you are someone who becomes attached to others easily. This allows you to love others freely, but there is the danger that you may cross over another's boundaries. Be sure that when you love people, you include yourself. A refusal to let go may indicate that you are operating out of fear.

REFLECT on what happens if you tighten your grip on the issue you've identified. Tighten the grip; hold on tighter and tighter. Soon something will break–and it may be you!

AFFIRM with feeling: "Today I release . . . in my life." Notice how you feel and what you think after doing this ritual.

SEI HEI KI MEDITATION

- You are in a hot-air balloon.
- There is an anchor holding you to earth even though you want very much to rise into the air. You look at the anchor and realize that it is composed of the thoughts and feelings that you've been holding on to even though they no longer serve you. You sit there for quite a while, wishing you could get off the ground. But the anchor of your attachment is holding you fast.
- Something strange is happening. There are seven balloons on the anchor. You know intuitively that you must release these balloons, one at a time, in order for your hot-air basket to rise up to freedom.
- Finally, after much soul-searching, you feel that maybe, just maybe, you might let go of one of the balloons. You choose the red one. You watch the red balloon float up and you feel yourself move up a tiny bit.
- You do the same thing with the orange balloon. You watch the orange balloon float up and you feel yourself move up a tiny bit more.
- Now the yellow balloon. You watch the yellow balloon float up and you feel yourself move up even more. This isn't too bad, you think. Now for the green one.

- The green balloon is harder to let go. It is your heart-space. It means a lot to you. But finally you let it go and you feel yourself move up quite a bit.
- You realize that there are three more balloons holding you just above the earth, blocking your flight into the sky where you know you will find freedom.
- A blue balloon floats in front of your eyes, held to the basket by a thin string of silver. As you release this balloon and watch it float away, your basket rises higher yet.
- Then you let go of an indigo balloon and rise higher.
- The only balloon left now is a purple one with a golden string. This is the hardest balloon of all to release. After a bit more deliberating and checking with your insides, you let go of it all and release the last balloon.
- Now you are free! Your hot-air balloon rises quickly and settles to a perfect height just right for you to see your entire life spread out below you. You are truly free! You know that you trust the Universe.

3. HARTH: LOVE AND COMPASSION

Is there enough love in your life? Are you receiving as well as giving? In what ways are you withholding love from yourself? In what ways are you withholding love from another?

Harth is the symbol for the heart from which healing and love flow. The heart is in the middle of the physical body. Harth means love, truth, beauty, harmony, and balance. The Harth symbol is not an original Reiki symbol. It was channeled by a Reiki master-teacher. Though it is not taught by all Reiki masters, it is widely accepted and loved by many Reiki practitioners and teachers. You may substitute the concept of Love for this symbol.

Harth speaks of Universal Love, not romantic love or erotic love. Universal Love is unconditional and flows freely throughout the Universe. With every inbreath you take, breathe in Love. With every outbreath that leaves your body, breathe out Love. The full exchange of Love energy will enrich and enhance your life.

The two polarities within this archetype are cherish and neglect. To cherish something or someone is to hold it dear to your heart. Caring is a quality vital to our human life. Yet when we care too much, we kill the very thing we love. Living things need freedom—freedom to grow, to change. We must be certain we are acting out of true caring for the well-being of the other, not from our own selfish interest. If we water a plant too much, it will die. If we keep it in the sun too long, it will not survive. If we plant a seed in the ground and then dig it up to see how it is doing, because we "cherish" it, the tiny roots will die. We must temper our caring with a healthy dose of loving neglect.

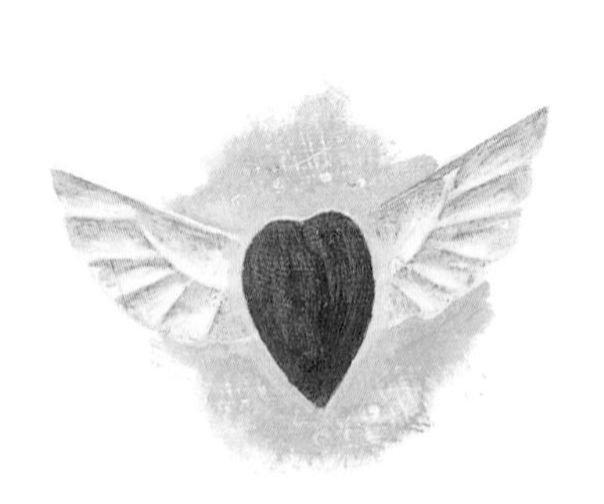

Neglect is at the opposite extreme of caring too much. Children who are completely neglected will not live. If we neglect to take care of something, it will not flourish. One of the things we often neglect is ourselves. A balance between caring too much for ourselves, being self-absorbed and disregarding our own needs, being irresponsible for our own well-being, is the balance we seek.

WHEN YOU DRAW THIS CARD you are being asked to examine your attitudes toward love in your life. Is there enough? Are you receiving as well as giving? In what ways are you withholding love from yourself? In what ways are you withholding love from another? Love is energy. Let it flow through you.

If the card is UPRIGHT, you are in the neighborhood of Cherishing. You care a great deal about others. You need to learn to cherish yourself as you do others. Notice whether you cherish another because you truly want what is good for him or her or because you want to control. You cannot control Love. It flows.

If the card is REVERSED, you may be neglecting an aspect of balanced Caring. Neglecting yourself by forgetting to take care of yourself is to be unbalanced, just as is being self-absorbed. Look at some of the ways in which you neglect yourself or someone you truly cherish. You cannot control by neglect.

REFLECT on ways in which you can allow love to freely flow throughout your being. As you sit quietly relaxed, become aware of your breathing. Breathe in and out, rhythmically and naturally, as the waves in the ocean move in and out, rhythmically and naturally. Rhythmic breathing is like pushing a swing high into the air. The upswing carries your love outward and then brings love back to you as it descends to the earth.

AFFIRM with feeling: "When I allow love to freely flow through me, I am energized and filled with Universal Love. I breathe love in and out."

HARTH MEDITATION

- Imagine yourself in a lovely park. It is a beautiful, warm spring day and you see a swing. You are tired and the swing looks very inviting, so you sit in it and begin to swing. Gently, slowly.
- Then you swing higher and higher. Now you feel someone invisible, a guardian angel, pushing the swing. The flow of the air increases as the swing gains momentum. You feel an intake of air as you are pulled backward and then, as you swing forward, high into the air, you feel the rush of air in the exhalation of your breath.

- The wind is the Breath of God. And the Breath of God carries Love to all parts of the Universe.
- As you swing forward, up into the air, you feel your love carried out into the world through your breath. As you swing backward toward the ground, you feel love returning to you through your breath.
- Your breath is the Breath of God. Breathe and Swing. Breathe and Swing.

4. HON SHA ZA SHO NEN: CONNECTION AND SERVICE

Forgive. Clear up a karmic debt. Serve.

Hon Sha Za Sho Nen is one of the original four Reiki symbols shown to Dr. Usui. It is one of the most powerful and universal symbols in the Reiki system. It means deep connection to others, near or distant. It means service to others. One translation of this symbol is, The Buddha (God) in me reaches out to the Buddha (God) in you to promote enlightenment and peace. Another translation is, I bestow the truth of truths upon you. As above, so below. As within, so without.

This is the symbol used for distant healing. When using this symbol, there is no past, no future, only the eternal now. All limitation is transcended. There is freedom from time, space, delusion, and limitation.

Whenever you send love, light, colors, prayer, or thoughts to someone and you imagine someone well, that is distant healing.

This symbol also implies forgiveness. We may use this principle to clear up a karmic debt.

The two polarities within this archetype are altruism and self-centeredness. Altruism is unselfish connection to others in the world. At this end of the continuum we find thoughts and behaviors that seem to have no ulterior motive, no hidden agenda. We must look to our motives in our interactions with others. It sounds good to think we are unselfish, but people who are totally unselfish often do not take responsibility for their own thoughts, feelings, and behavior. They can often blame others or themselves.

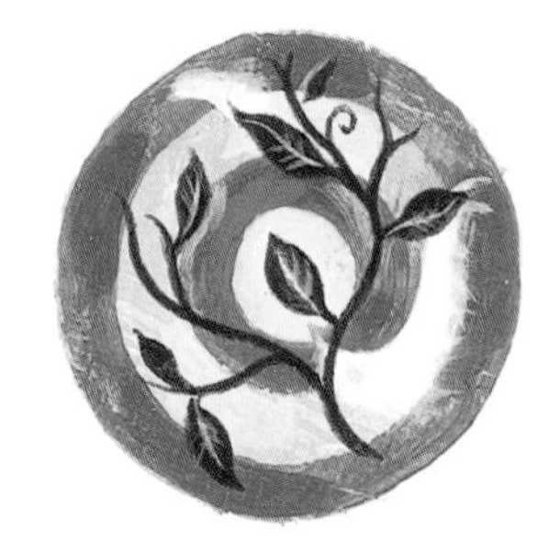

By contrast, when we are self-centered, we disconnect ourselves from other people. We become "self-ish." We cannot be of service to the world if we are disconnected. We cannot serve the world if we disconnect from ourselves and our own essence. We need to evaluate this principle situation by situation. Each one is unique. We must clarify our intent. For example, we may appear to be selfish by backing off when someone doesn't really need our help. If we don't "help" those who don't need help, we may be strengthening them by forcing them to take responsibility when it's appropriate.

WHEN YOU DRAW THIS CARD you are being asked to reach out to someone who is physically or emotionally distant from you. Mentally and emotionally stretch your spirit out and ask if this person's Higher Self wants you to send Reiki (love) energy. If the answer is yes, send your prayers and your love and your healing energy. Follow your intuition on this matter and, most important, let go of the outcome.

If the card is UPRIGHT, it may look as if you are acting in an unselfish manner, but only you know your inner motives. Examine your intent and be sure you feel a deep connection with others at the soul level.

If the card is REVERSED, you may be unwilling to forgive someone or be holding on to a past hurt for selfish reasons. Examine your intent.

REFLECT on those you've become estranged from, either physically, mentally, or emotionally. Think about the ways in which you might judge other people or yourself. Think about ways in which you might release the energy bound up in judgment and nonforgiveness. Write a letter to yourself or to another and ask forgiveness for your own transgression.

AFFIRM with feeling: "I send this love and healing to [person's name] for his or her soul's highest purpose."

HON SHA ZA SHO NEN MEDITATION

- Imagine that you are part of a giant stained-glass mosaic. Every living thing in the world is also a facet of the mosaic. In addition, each facet of the mosaic is a hologram, so that each person's entire life is contained in the facet.
- The mosaic is a living, breathing organism, like the earth. The effect of this is that everything you do affects and is affected by others.
- Imagine now that as you inhale oxygen, you are breathing in the energy of those around you, even those at the far end of the mosaic. As you move through your life, you are very respectful of what you do. You are very careful and mindful of your place in the giant mosaic of the world.

5. ZONAR: PAST LIVES AND ANCESTOR REVERENCE

Examine your relations with your family of origin. Ask your parents or siblings about your ancestors (grandparents, great-grandparents) and ask them for help. They may be your spirit guides.

Zonar is not an original Reiki symbol but was "found" by a Reiki master at a later date.

It means infinity, timelessness, eternity. This symbol works well for past-life, karmic issues. In the Archetypal Reiki system, it stands for family love and loyalty and ancestor work.

Often there is a persistent problem area in your life that just doesn't seem to have any roots in your own past or in any other source that you know of. Perhaps this is a past-life issue, an issue of karma. *Karma* is a sanskrit word for action, for cause and effect, for balance.

The two polarities of this archetype are belonging and alienation. Honoring our ancestors and family love and loyalty are part of the principle of belonging. We are born into a family. Within that family we learn the rules of conduct appropriate for the culture to which we belong. If we have learned maladaptive rules and customs, we need to reexamine these in the light of our adult life. When we are growing up, we often want to belong so much to a particular group that we give up our own ethical system and take on the norms of the group. When the group is healthy, this works well. If the group is unhealthy, we are in trouble. We cannot sacrifice everything in order to belong. Too much time spent at this end of the continuum results in ethnocentricity and a "we-they" mentality—that is, "we" are always right; "they" are always wrong.

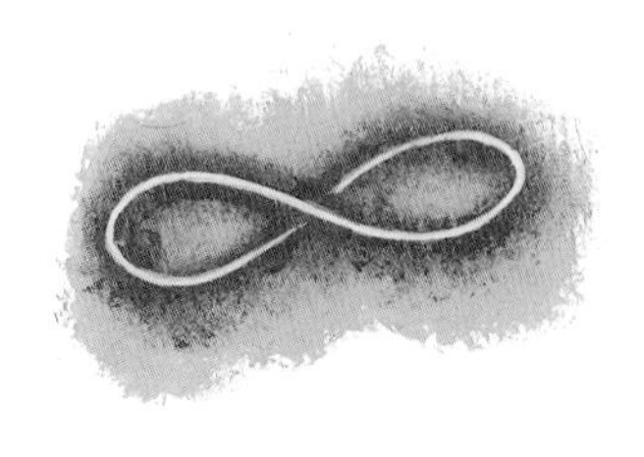

At the other end of the spectrum is alienation. If we move away inappropriately from our family of origin, or do not adhere to the norms of our healthy group, we become alienated and isolated. We live on the fringes of our society and often we are alienated from ourselves as well. This results in having no clearly defined ethical system; no standards to refer our behavior to. We are lost. A healthy balance between false loyalty and inner or outer isolation is the key to this archetype.

WHEN YOU DRAW THIS CARD in a reading, contemplate the meaning of time and its other dimensions. You are being asked to examine your relations with your family of origin.

What is it in your life that does not seem traceable to your personal history but which you may have been "born with"? Think about this and put your answers in your journal. You may want to do a Reiki card reading on this topic also. Shuffle your deck and split it into two piles. Formulate your question and draw one card from the pile on your left; then draw another card from the pile on your right for an answer. From the answer, formulate another question. Continue this process until you feel finished. This will result in a dialogue with your inner guidance on this issue.

If the card is UPRIGHT, you have good feelings of belonging to your social groups. If there are any fences to mend in your family or among your family of choice, your friends, do it this week.

If the card is REVERSED, you may be feeling alienated from yourself or not in touch with your deepest roots. You may want to go to a cemetery and visit some of your loved ones who have traveled beyond the veil. Talk to them. They may help.

AFFIRM with feeling: "When I use the word *zonar* I have the intention to heal anything with which I may have come into this world. I ask my familial ancestors to please help in this healing."

ZONAR MEDITATION

- Go into the hallway of your mind. There you will find a set of ten stone steps. Slowly count backward from ten to one. As you descend the stairway, you come into a white mist. Soon the white mist surrounds and envelops you. You feel safe and comfortable in this place.
- In front of you is a doorway. You feel compelled to open the door and enter. As you

enter, the white mist disappears and you find yourself at a long table filled with the objects and situations of your current life.

- Examine these items, then pick out the one that is most disturbing to you. You need an answer to a question. Write the question in black marker on a large white board. Picture the situation that is troubling you. As you watch, the white mist again fills the room.
- When the mist clears, you find yourself in the life in which this problem originated. Watch and see what happens.
- Go back the same way you came in. This time, as you ascend the stairs, slowly count from one to ten. Journal your experience.

6. DAI KO MYO: SPIRITUAL HEALING

All healing has a spiritual root cause. Attend to your health at the spiritual level.

Dai Ko Myo (pronounced day-ko-me-o) is one of the four original symbols that Dr. Usui saw on the mountain. It is the highest of all the Reiki symbols. The person using this symbol does healing for the sake of others, with pure intent.

There are two forms of Dai Ko Myo. One is the traditional Japanese-Tibetan symbol that was given to Dr. Usui. The other has been channeled by Reiki master Diane Stein (author of *Essential Reiki*). In Archetypal Reiki Healing work, Dai Ko Myo is used as a mantra.

The opposing forces within this archetype are awakening and sleep-trance. Being awake is a state of consciousness in which we are fully and completely aware that we are spiritual beings in human form and we are all One. If a person were able to live at this end of the continuum, he or she would be an ascended master. Ascended masters are those who have achieved enlightenment and have passed through the veil (died to earthly concerns). If we lived here, we would not need to be in human form at all. We are allowed a glimpse of this state of spirit when we see through the personalities of ourselves and those around us and relate at the soul level. We could not live on the earthly plane if we did this always.

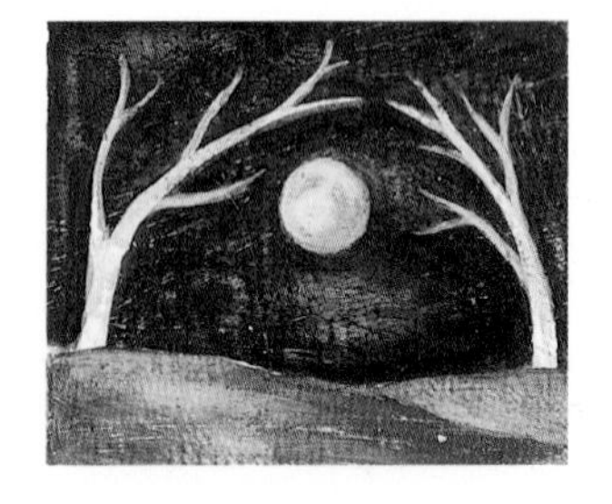

On the other end of the spectrum are those of us who live perpetually in a light trance, the trance of the "walking dead." In this state, we have no recognition of our spirituality at all and we think that the material world of our five senses is all there is. Most people move into this trance when there are repetitive, meaningless tasks to do. We call it being "on automatic pilot." We become "numbed out." We cannot live too much or too long at this end.

We need to move along toward the middle, where we can see the bright light of awakening and feel much rejoicing in spiritual matters yet still have recognition, acceptance, and appreciation of our human nature.

WHEN YOU DRAW THIS CARD in a reading it is time to do a daily Dai Ko Myo healing for yourself. Find a point on each shoulder blade, in the bony hollow of the back. Massage the point on one shoulder with the fingertips of the opposite hand. Use a clockwise motion. When you are finished, make a loose fist and lightly tap on your chest just above the breastbone about fifteen times. Although the thymus has atrophied in adulthood, this exercise will stimulate the heart chakra. The entire exercise is valuable for your immune system.

If the card is UPRIGHT, you are aware and awake to your spirituality. Be sure your spiritual practice is in place on a daily basis. It may be that you live too much at the top of your head—that is, in the spirit world. In this case, you may be ignoring important emotions. Move closer to the middle so that your spirituality can be acted out through your body.

If the card is REVERSED, you may often be in a trance. This means that you have learned to dissociate your attention from your physical reality. If you live here too long or too often, you will not be conscious enough to do the work necessary for spiritual development.

AFFIRM with feeling: "I ask for healing at the spiritual root of all dis-ease. My immune system is strong and healthy."

DAI KO MYO MEDITATION

- You find a silver door. Move through the door into your body. Move into one organ system at a time. Go through the emotions you've been feeling lately. Now go into your mind. Move through the thoughts you've been thinking lately. Do not become attached to anything you experience.
- In the hallway of your mind you will find a golden door, and you will feel compelled to enter that door. Reach out and turn the golden knob. As you walk through the golden door you see all around you a world of spirits. You are yourself in spirit form. When you look at your own spirit, you notice that there are some dark spots within the light that is you. As you examine the dark spots, you find in one your lack of faith in God and the spirit world. You don't seem to have the confidence

you once had that all will be well. You feel dismayed by your lack of faith and determine to do something about it.

- You approach a special altar that is in the spirit world. Upon the altar is a vase of beautiful, fresh, sweet-smelling flowers and a key. The flowers are to remind you that you are of the earth and that, like the beautiful flowers, you will one day be recycled.
- You pick up the key and know deep within yourself that this is the key to your heart. You place the key over your heart and intone this prayer: "Although I often move through a dark, frightening valley, I have willingness in my heart to open to Your Love. It is at the times of greatest blindness that I move in faith. I vow this day to keep moving, even though I cannot see my way on the path. I trust Your Light and Love will keep me warm and safe. Thank you."

7. REIKI: SPIRITUALLY DIRECTED HEALING

Reiki energy goes where it is needed, bringing all levels of existence—body, mind, heart, and spirit—into balance, into harmony.

Reiki (pronounced ray-key) is the name Dr. Usui gave to his "way of natural healing." (In Japan it would be pronounced lay-key, since there is no "r" sound in Japanese.) *Reiki* means Universal Energy (Godmind) merging with life force energy (human consciousness).

The two poles within this archetype are wholeness and fragmentation. When we operate at the wholeness end of the continuum, we may think we have the "whole picture" when what we really have is another gestalt (a configuration so unified that its parts cannot be separated out). When we get new or different information, our whole gestalt is shattered, only to be re-formed into yet another whole picture. This is how we learn. It is possible that only God sees "the whole."

Or we may see a whole picture that is erroneous. Old ideas, old concepts, old notions are often accepted as absolutes when they may not be working any longer. We must not get complacent and smug about our wholeness. Move over a little.

At the other end is fragmentation. To be fragmented is painful, yet it takes the breaking up of old patterns for new forms to emerge. It takes chaos for creation to occur. The seeds of the beginning are in the ending. When our dreams have been shattered, when we feel fragmented, we must hold on to one thing that is stable in our lives and know that unconscious forces are working to create yet another wholeness.

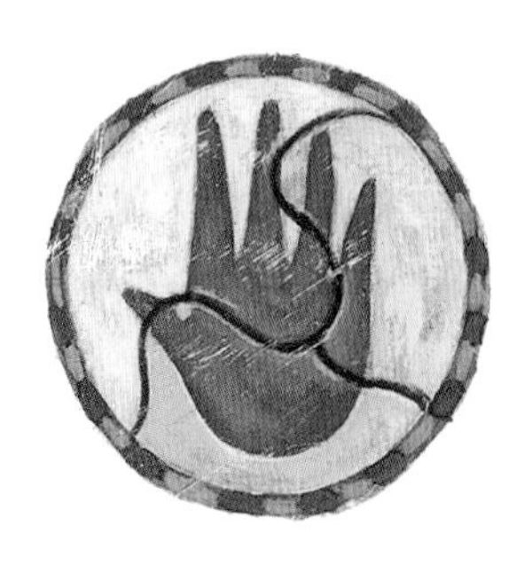

WHEN YOU DRAW THIS CARD you must allow the Reiki energy to enter your being. Feel the ki flowing in your body-mind-soul. Send out your ki to someone who is in need.

If the card is UPRIGHT, you know that your ki is flowing easily and naturally throughout your system.

If the card is REVERSED, there may be a blockage somewhere. Scan your body-mind to see where you feel blocked. You will know intuitively where you are stuck.

AFFIRM with feeling: "I honor my holy ki and I practice allowing the Reiki energy to flow within my self and to others, with love and respect."

REIKI MEDITATION

- You are seated before a mirror. The mirror is reflecting someone. You think it must be you. It is you, but an otherworldly you. The best that is you, your highest essence.
- You recognize the reflection before you as your Higher Self. Your Higher Self holds the symbol for rei in his or her right hand and the symbol for ki in his or her left hand. See the symbols in front of you. Notice the color, the shape, and then reach out and touch the symbols. Notice how they feel.
- Your Higher Self holds rei above your head, just above your crown chakra. Instantly you feel the most wonderful, awesome love and warmth and comfort and peace, as if it is raining soft stardust filled with love, warmth, comfort, peace upon your head.
- This Sacred Rain comes through your head and fills your entire body with its silver light and love.
- Your Higher Self now holds ki to your bare feet and, instantly, you feel a surge of powerful, liquid fire move through your feet up your body, filling your entire body with tremendous energy and vitality, such as you have never before felt.
- Filled with the miraculous healing Reiki energy, you return to your meditation spot, and you carry this energy with you throughout your day.

8. SEARCH FOR TRUTH: PILGRIMAGE

A search for your truth involves complete emotional and spiritual honesty about the events in your life. Do a self-inventory of your part in creating the situation you are in.

The search for Truth is represented by the founder of Reiki, Mikao Usui. Dr. Usui was not satisfied with less than authenticity in healing, and so he made a difficult pilgrimage to the holy mountain to learn how to heal. While there he was given the Truth of Reiki healing. Modeling ourselves after Dr. Usui, we each must embark on our own pilgrimage so that we can live a genuine life of authenticity.

The polarities within this archetype are authenticity and denial. An authentic person lives by standards or criteria he or she has found to be true and real. One problem with living completely at this end of the spectrum is that you may become convinced that there is only one Truth. You must learn, however, to accept the Truth of others and to love the authentic self of others, even though you may not "like" it. We must learn to search for the Truth as Reiki's founder did, and to look beneath the surface for the meaning of what is happening.

By contrast, when we live in denial, we are living the Lie. We refuse to accept the truth in our situation. We refuse to accept flaws and imperfections in ourselves or others. We will not acknowledge our human nature as being less than perfect. The most important part of truth-telling is that we tell ourselves the truth as we see it. Truth is not only telling the truth; it is living the Truth in a most authentic, genuine, real way.

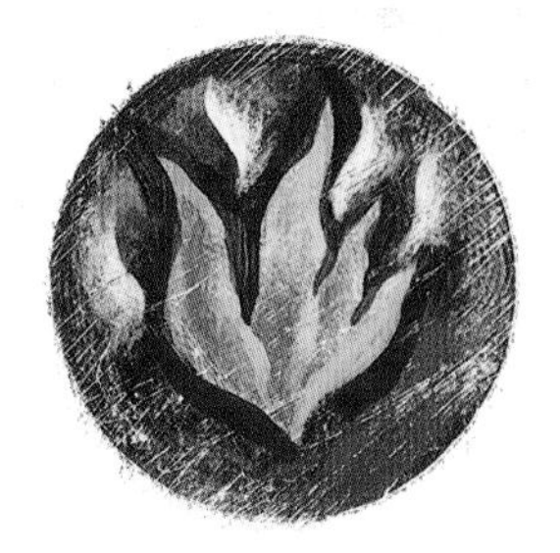

WHEN YOU DRAW THIS CARD in a reading you have the honor of receiving the blessings of Dr. Usui. You have been on your own quest for Truth. The pilgrimage for Truth can be made either physically or through meditation and visualization.

If the card is UPRIGHT, you are ready and willing to examine your life and take responsibility for changing what you do not like.

If the card is REVERSED, you need to become more emotionally honest. This means you need to face what you may be in denial about. Being spiritually honest means looking at the times you say "I can't" when you mean "I won't."

AFFIRM with feeling: "The truth I seek is the Holy Truth. It is my truth."

SEARCH FOR TRUTH MEDITATION

- In preparation for your journey to Truth, ask the spirit of Dr. Usui to be with you and to guide you. Set the time for your journey, and for a month (or a year) before that time eat nourishing foods; drink clear, clean water; exercise your physical body so you will have the endurance for your journey—and to make your body sacred.
- Go to the desert, a mountain, an ocean, a forest—or any other place you feel is a sacred power spot on the earth. Find your sacred waterfall.
- Drop your "robes of the city." As you step into the rainbow waterfall, allow any and all negative feelings to leave your body. Bring to mind feelings of guilt, shame, fear, disappointment, betrayal, and despair and allow the healing waters to wash them away into the earth, where they are neutralized.
- As negative thoughts come to mind, allow the healing waterfall to wash them all clean: "You're not good enough. There is not enough [time, money, health, friends, love]." Watch the negative thoughts flow down the mountainside and into the pool of God's love, where they are neutralized.
- Any lack in your life is healed now. No one can hurt or damage you. The rainbow waterfall cleanses, purifies, and carries away any and all sickness of spirit you feel inside. You feel refreshed, re-created, and renewed. You release everything from your past and become willing to begin again.
- Putting on fresh, clean robes and new shoes, and bringing enough fresh food and clean water to last the duration of your trip, you start out for your destination.
- The next part of your journey takes place when you arrive at the mountain. Begin the long, arduous ascent up the spiritual mountain. When you are halfway up you pass the point of no return and you realize that you are now committed, for better

or worse, to this path. Climb up and up, through all the storms and different weathers of the mountain.

- As you walk, release more and more of the thoughts and feelings and spiritual dread from your past. Know that you are severing your past, irrevocably. Become more and more empty.
- At the top of the mountain you see the sun in all its glory. Feel the life-giving warmth and the healing rays of the sun. At this peak moment in your spiritual journey, sit down and make a ritual of gratitude.
- For twenty-one days, you fast, meditate, pray, and contemplate the nature of Truth.
- At the end of that time you are given a spectacular gift. The gift is your Truth. It may appear in symbolic form or it may be a concrete object or idea.
- Drop the lie and hear your Truth now.
- Write the Truth in your journal and live authentically with the Truth in your heart.
- Return to your community, bringing your Truth with you to share with those you love and those you influence. Celebrate and rejoice, for you have returned with more than what you left with.

9. REIKI IDEALS: EMOTIONAL DISCIPLINE

The Reiki ideals are a prescription for how to live with utter grace and abundance. Feel the abundance around you.

After his spiritual experience on Mount Kuriyama, Dr. Usui began to work with the Reiki healing energy. He then developed five ideals for "the secret art of inviting happiness." All five ideals revolve around a belief in living in the present moment, the now. They are usually written in English like this:

Just for today, do not anger.
Just for today, do not worry.
Just for today, work hard (interpreted as meditative practice).
Just for today, be kind to every living thing.
Just for today, be grateful.

The two extremes of this archetype are equanimity and over/underreaction. When we repress our emotions, we become sick physically, emotionally, or spiritually. When we live at this end of the continuum, we do not even acknowledge or recognize our emotions, let alone express them. Anger, worry, and feelings of scarcity will be acted out if we do not acknowledge and express them or if we are prone to the emotional outbursts that injure everyone around us, and ourselves, and we do nothing to solve the problem. We must move to the center and express our emotions appropriately, realistically, and with care.

Equanimity or emotional discipline is not obedience or punishment. Discipline, instead, is training. Emotions can be trained to serve our spirituality. If our emotions are not disciplined or trained, we become confused about spiritual principles in our lives. Once we have our emotions in hand, we are free to develop ourselves spiritually.

WHEN YOU DRAW THIS CARD in a reading you are advised to observe your behavior for the next week. See how often you are able to live in the moment, in the now. Notice whether you are living in some past that you can't let go of, or in some future that you can't control.

If the card is UPRIGHT, you tend to swallow your feelings and often do not know how you feel at any given time. You are slow to express your feelings and this can get you in trouble with those closest to you.

If the card is REVERSED, you probably victimize yourself and others with your emotional outbursts. You may feel in control and even powerful when you do this, but it's a short-lived and unhealthy form of controlling those around you. Move toward the center.

REFLECT on whether your emotions are in alignment with your soul. Soul is soft and gentle in her responses to others and to herself. If you are excessive or inhibited in any of the ways described in the five ideals, you are being asked to change your response. Reflection on abundance will help you. Try this: There is a simple way to align with the life force so as to feel the abundance around you. Stand for three minutes, feet apart, arms and hands outstretched, left palm up and right palm down. The ki energy surrounding you enters your left palm and flows through the heart and solar plexus, charging your entire body, with the surplus flowing out through your right hand.

Morning will bring a surge of energy; evening will bring relaxation. Now focus your entire attention on being successful in all you do and abundant in all you are.

AFFIRM with feeling: "Just for today, I am peaceful, calm, kind, devoted, and grateful for all the abundance in my life."

REIKI IDEALS MEDITATION

- You are going on a special journey, a journey of love and peace. You are going to a special, spiritual mountain far away. It is to be a long and arduous trip on which you will encounter many obstacles and difficulties. You must be well prepared and well rested in order to undertake such a journey of truth.
- Just before you embark, you realize that you are carrying five bags. In fact, it seems to you that you've always carried these bags. Then you get the inner guidance that it is time to open these bags and see what is inside.
- You open them one at a time. In the first bag you find your anger. All the strong

anger, smoldering resentments, bitter disappointments, small irritations that have grown big over time, and wrathful rage bent on vengeance are in this bag. You make the conscious decision to empty this bag. You find a cliff and toss the contents of the bag, followed by the bag itself, over the side. You feel a little lighter. But there are four more bags.

- You open the second bag and inside you see all your petty worries, your immobilizing fears, your nagging concerns that have grown over the years into big fears and guilts. You make a conscious decision to empty the bag over another cliff. As you throw the bag over the cliff, you release all the fears that have been holding you back. You feel a lot lighter.
- In the third bag you find your reluctance to meditate properly and consistently. You find, inside this bag, your distractions, your idle chatter, your laziness, and all the other things that keep you from your Source. You quickly, without thinking, toss the entire bag over another cliff.
- There is a fourth bag to deal with now. In this bag you find all the living things, including parts of yourself, that you have been unkind to, disrespectful of, or have dishonored due to your own carelessness. All of these living things are weeping. You weep, too, as you take them out, one by one, and you caress and hold them, murmuring your regrets.
- As they each feel better, they scamper off to where they belong; no longer are they confined by your unkindness to them. You feel so much better and so much lighter, you think you can move on now. But something is holding you back. The final bag.
- This, of course, is your bag of ingratitude. In it you find all of your complaints, your self-pity, your beliefs in scarcity. You fill this bag with gratitude for the abundance you've been given and leave the bag open for another person to find. You are now free and joyous to continue your journey to the mountain. Peace and love follow you. Amen.

10. INTENT AND PURPOSE: PURITY AND CLARITY

Reflect on the metaphysical law that what you send out returns to you tenfold. You are not asked to be perfect, only vigilant.

Intent and Purpose, as well as Desire, form the basis for any spiritual discipline and are necessary for all healing to take place. When utilizing the Reiki healing energy, it is our intention and purpose that allows the Reiki energy to flow freely.

It is said that when God created the world out of its own energy, with intent and purpose, the deed was done. We are part of that God-Power. We are cocreators. We must cocreate with great humility, respect, and responsibility.

The polarities within this archetype are purity-clarity and purposelessness. We cannot live as if we have absolutely pure intent and absolute clarity of purpose. We are human beings, and to act as if we are perfect is living a lie. We must, however, strive to keep ourselves as uncontaminated as possible. We need to move toward the middle of this continuum.

At this end of the spectrum, chaos, ill will, and purposelessness exist side by side. But we cannot accept this as our norm. If everything is chaotic, we ourselves may be creating the chaos. Even though not all chaos is negative, we cannot live here all of the time. Chaos comes before creation, so if things seem chaotic, there may be a beautiful light at the other end.

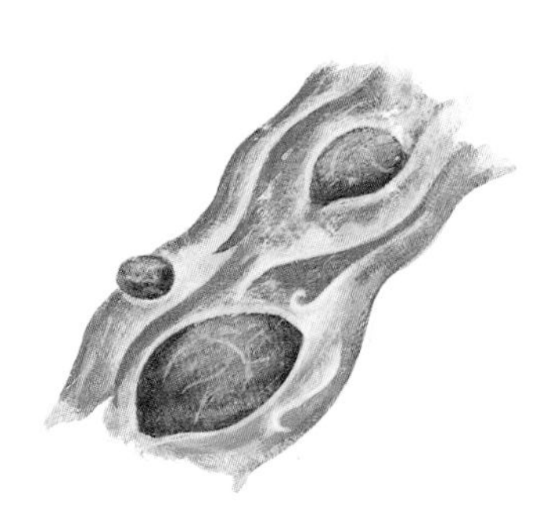

If all is random chance and nothing matters anyway, there is no purpose to our lives and we may become depressed and despondent. We must watch our intent and move toward the center. We must seek balance.

WHEN YOU DRAW THIS CARD in a reading you are asked to examine your motives to be sure that your intents are not contaminated with your own greed, and that what you desire is in the interests of your soul's highest purpose.

If the card is UPRIGHT, you are acting with reasonably pure intention and your purpose is in alignment with the soul's highest purpose.

If the card is REVERSED, you may be contaminating the healing situation with your own agenda. Examine your motives more deeply.

AFFIRM with feeling: "I ask that my intentions be pure and my purpose clear. May this healing take place for the good of our soul's highest purpose and that of Mother Earth."

INTENT AND PURPOSE MEDITATION

- You are a deep bowl, ready to receive guidance from the Reiki masters and teachers.
- You are in a room filled with the clear white light of Spirit. The white light is radiating love and healing from the most beatific being on earth. Within the light you clearly see the purpose of your Archetypal Reiki work.
- Into the bowl that is you falls pure, clean water from the Cosmic Mountain of your dreams. The water and the light are clear, pure, free of hidden desires, and uncluttered by earthly attachments.
- Although you don't consciously "know" your soul's highest purpose, you are glad to be a vehicle through which your soul can act out its purpose. You thank the Source for the gifts you have received through Archetypal Reiki work.

11. GROUNDING AND BALANCE: FOUNDATION

Consider ways in which you might be out of balance. Only when we are grounded—rooted in sensation, feeling, action, and in the solidity of the material world—can we heal.

Grounding is an important principle in all energy work. Balance is the goal of all spiritual practice. When we give or receive Reiki, our energy system is automatically balanced: if we are too "cold," Reiki will warm us; if we are too "warm," Reiki will cool us.

Our major energy pathways run vertically through our bodies, while subtler currents run in other directions. This earth-centered pole keeps us connected to the earth and in balance with the natural world in which we live. When energetic contact is made through the body, it is called grounding. Grounding means we are conscious that our body is connected to the earth, and it comes from the solid contact we make with the earth through our feet and legs. Any excess energy is discharged down into the ground. We feel, then, that we can stand on our own two feet and move forward in life.

Only when we are grounded can we be present, focused, and dynamic. Only when we are rooted in sensation, feeling, action, and in the solidity of the material world can we begin to raise our consciousness. When consciousness is detached from the body, it is too wide, vague, and empty to be useful to our spiritual development. When consciousness is connected to our body, we have a dynamic energy flow throughout our entire being. We have "plugged in" the system.

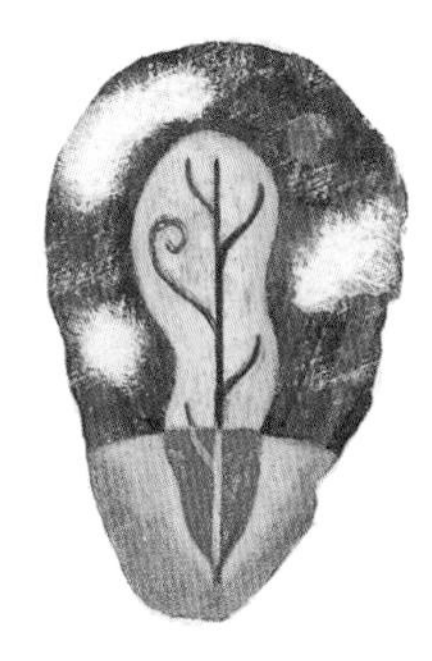

The polarities within this archetype are centered and scattered. When we are centered, we feel whole and complete. We need to be able to respond to the world around us and not ignore its legitimate calls. When we are centered, we have a centerpoint, and we know where it is and how to get there. When we get offbalance from the stresses and strains of everyday life, we know how to become centered again in a healthy way.

When our energy is scattered, we don't accomplish much and we are in a constant state of upheaval. When a trauma occurs, our energy will become scattered, and if the situation goes on too long, we may even become fragmented. We cannot live in a state of chronic crisis; problems must be resolved if we are to return to our center. With God as our center, we need not fear. Move closer to the other end.

WHEN YOU DRAW THIS CARD in a reading you are offbalance in some way. Maybe a life trauma has hurt you and spread your energy around. You need to do a ritual to be in harmony again.

If the card is UPRIGHT, you are centered much of the time. Keep yourself that way. Be sure you're also in touch with Mother Earth physically.

If the card is REVERSED, you need equilibrium in your life. You may need to do an exercise to ground you again. Try this: Stand with your feet shoulder-width apart, hands at sides. Find the center of your body by rocking gently from side to side and from front to back until you feel a stillpoint. Imagine yourself to be an oak tree, your roots connected to the earth with branches reaching to the sky. Carry this feeling with you for the next week.

AFFIRM with feeling: "I am firmly connected to the ground of Mother Earth. I am balanced in my life."

GROUNDING AND BALANCE MEDITATION

- You are seated at a table in a place familiar to you. On the table is a large jigsaw puzzle depicting the significant parts of your life. The picture is not complete; some pieces are missing. In the picture, you see the times in your life when the wind of Spirit blew through you; the times you walked through the dark tunnel with no end; the times you fell to the bottom of the bottomless pit; the times you fell in love—with a person and with life itself. It's all there.
- You sit there, reliving the parts, contemplating, thinking about what it all means. You feel some urgency about coming to peace with yourself.
- Suddenly, a door opens and a strong wind blows through the room, scattering the

pieces of your puzzle. Scattering the pieces of your life all over the floor. You frantically try to pick them all up, but the wind blows more strongly now. Your heart drops as you try to fight the wind of change.

- You try for a long time to pick up the scattered pieces. For days, weeks, months, and even years. You wail. You rage. You pray. You logically try to figure out which pieces go where. You ask the opinions of others. Nothing works! You are soul-sick.
- Finally, you surrender to what is. You surrender to what will be. You sit down in the middle of the mess your life has become. You bow your head in surrender and you weep. As your tears fall, you slip into that quiet, sacred place deep within you.
- A strong wind comes up again, only this time the wind comes from that place deep within yourself. The scattered pieces of your life fall into place and you see the whole picture. No fragments. You laugh. You laugh long and loud.

12. PRAYER AND MEDITATION: OPENING AND CLOSING

Examine the ways in which you pray. Try letting thoughts and feelings of love and appreciation flow through your being. That is prayer and meditation.

Prayer and meditation are the foundation of all spiritual disciplines. Prayer is opening yourself to your higher consciousness in an active way. There are as many forms of prayer as there are human needs. These range from the solitary, quiet, contemplative prayer without much form to formal recitations, verbal exercises, and specific imagery. It has been said that an essential ingredient in making prayer "work" is love–compassion, empathy, and deep caring. The kind of love that releases and is not invested in the outcome.

Meditation connects us with our deepest self and with our Source. It creates a space within us so that Spirit can enter and allows transformation to take place. Of all the practices, meditation is the strongest way to a change in consciousness. In meditation we try to get past the control of our conscious mind. We allow ourselves to relax and the fragmented parts of us to coalesce and become whole.

The polarities within this archetype are openness to divine communication and a closed heart. When our hearts are open to love and our souls are open to God, we are in a place full of grace. A place of giving and receiving. We give to God and we give to the god within another person. But when we give to another with an open heart, we make ourselves vulnerable. We give another person the power to hurt us or to help us. The caution here is that we do not hold ourselves open to negative forces in the material world or the spirit world. We ask for protection and we examine our motives.

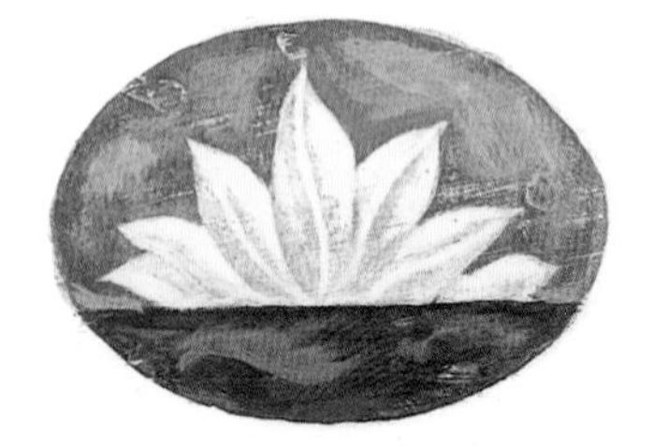

Giving can be a form of control if we are too open, too extreme. If we give our love to God, there is no guarantee that our material lives will be perfect. If we give our love to another, there is no guarantee that we will not be hurt, for it is part of human nature to take advantage of another's generosity.

If, on the other hand, we are too frightened or too angry to give with our hearts, we remain closed to any blessings or grace we might receive. A closed heart protects the one inside and keeps out danger, but it also keeps out love and abundance.

Balance is the key in this archetype, as it is in all Archetypal Reiki. We need to learn to give and receive as an exchange of energy.

WHEN YOU DRAW THIS CARD in a reading you are being asked to examine the ways in which you pray. You may be praying like a child, asking for something daily, as if God is Santa Claus.

If the card is UPRIGHT, the energy that is your prayer is truly thoughts given or sent with love and deep caring. You are open to divine communication in the form of sending or receiving.

If the card is REVERSED, you are too distracted when you meditate and too greedy when you pray. Look to your intent when you pray or meditate. Listen quietly. Open your heart.

Let your prayer flow through you. Pray from love, not from fear. Pray from soul, not from ego. Pray from the heart, not from the head. Pray in the present tense, as if it has already happened. Try "Let me be a clear channel for your love."

AFFIRM with feeling: "Today I create a prayer that is from my soul and I meditate upon the gifts I have been given."

PRAYER AND MEDITATION MEDITATION

- You are filled with openness to the Divine. Your heart is not a closed place, but is filled with the light of the divine within.
- You stand facing east. The sun is just coming up. It fills the sky with the pink-purple of its magnificence. You are filled with awe as you behold the majesty of nature. You raise your hands to the sky with open palms facing upward. As you watch the sun rise above the clouds, your spirit rises to its fullest and stands in awesome reverence.
- You give out all the love and beauty that is yours to give. And then you listen. You bow your head and you listen in quiet meditation for the voice of Spirit to enter your soul. Hear the message. Heed the message that you hear.

13. TRUST INNER GUIDANCE, IN REIKI AND IN SELF

Repeat this affirmation throughout the week: I will keep myself honorable and respectful to myself and to others. I will keep my life open to change and growth.

Hawayo Takata was made the first woman Reiki master when, following her own inner guidance, she traveled on faith and trust to Tokyo for her healing. She was also very diversified in the ways that she taught Reiki and did Reiki treatments. She taught that diversity is to be valued. Even though we are all different, we can all learn to trust. Without basic trust, all is lost.

Within this archetype are the two poles of trust and cynicism. If we trust the Universe, we also trust our Selves, especially our Higher Selves. To trust means to have faith, to have confidence that events in our lives have meaning and often work out "for the best." The "best" may be our soul's highest purpose rather than our ego's need. We do not need to become cynical in order to live with balance.

The opposite of trust is cynicism. The cynic is often a bitter, angry person who always maintains control. This is a person who believes that everyone is motivated by pure selfishness. And that there is, in fact, no Higher Power whose love motivates us. To trust is to let go of control, and the cynic cannot afford to do that, for then he or she will be abandoned in a cold, cruel world.

While it is true that most ideas need to be carefully examined to see whether they hold merit, we must not go to the extreme in mistrusting. We do not need to become a cynic, but we do need to evaluate objectively some things and some people. If we consistently mistrust, we do not honor and respect anything or anyone and often hold others in contempt for their perceived base motives. We can learn to live in harmony with both evaluation and trust in our hearts.

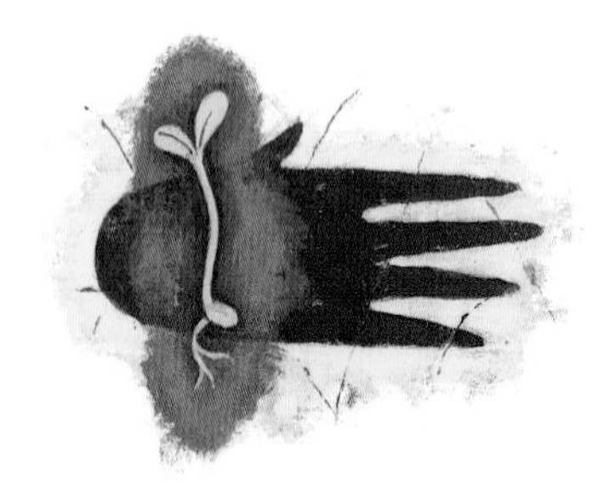

WHEN YOU DRAW THIS CARD in a reading you may have had to turn personal tragedy into a healing situation. You have been able to trust, respect, and honor all traditions, even if they differ from your own.

If the card is UPRIGHT, you are working well with the idea of trusting your own inner guidance. You are also learning to trust Archetypal Reiki.

If the card is REVERSED, you may be expressing an inner mistrust of yourself and of the Universe that is undeserved. Examine your motives.

REFLECT on the ways in which you express yourself. Ask for feedback from a dear or close friend as to how you are coming across in your communications. Ask if you are seen as a trustworthy person by others.

TRUST MEDITATION

- You have become a giant being. You are bigger than the earth. You are a shaman, capable of shifting shape at will. You travel all around the earth and even into the earth, observing all manner of life and nonlife upon the earth.
- You change form and you are an eagle, wings spread and clear-eyed, able to see the smallest speck under your body.
- You see a small rabbit and you become a rabbit. Your nose wrinkles and your ears elongate. The rabbit runs from the tiger. Your body becomes long and lean. You have claws that dig into trees for climbing. You stalk your prey and . . .
- You see an elephant calmly drinking from a cool mountain stream. Your nose becomes a trunk as you pull food into your mouth.
- There is a rock, a mountain. You become still and hard. You are stone.
- Now you are huge and high. You are a mountain.
- In rapid succession, you become a tree and then you are a forest of trees.
- You move through the oceans of the world and become a whale, the largest mammal on earth. You observe the myriad and differing forms of life in the sea. Fish, coral, seaweed, sand on the beaches.
- You now see the millions of insects and other tiny, microscopic forms of life and nonlife around you, from the smallest dust mite to the largest of the insect world.
- When you have traveled all over the world, the thing you are most struck by is the amazing diversity of all life and nonlife. There is order in the Universe. You deeply respect and honor all of the Universe. You trust the Universe in its order.

14. TRANSCENDENCE: SACRED SURRENDER

Act for the common good. Your sacrifice will be made sacred through clear purpose and pure intention.

Dr. Chujiro Hayashi, Dr. Usui's successor, showed us the meaning of sacrifice made sacred when he created his own transition (made himself die) rather than betray the Reiki ideals and traditions. So, too, we must learn to sacrifice unworthy qualities such as pride, arrogance, or greed, in order to live a life of transcendence.

The opposing forces within this archetype are transcendence or surrender and defeat or holding tight. To transcend means to pass beyond a human limit. To live in this sphere all the time is not humanly possible, nor is it desirable. To surrender our will to the will of God is a spiritual goal, but we cannot avoid responsibility for our own human actions and our own human life. We surrender our will and transcend our lower human selves only after we have done all that is humanly possible to remedy a particular situation. In this way, we have done our part and have fulfilled our covenant to move into spirituality through our material world.

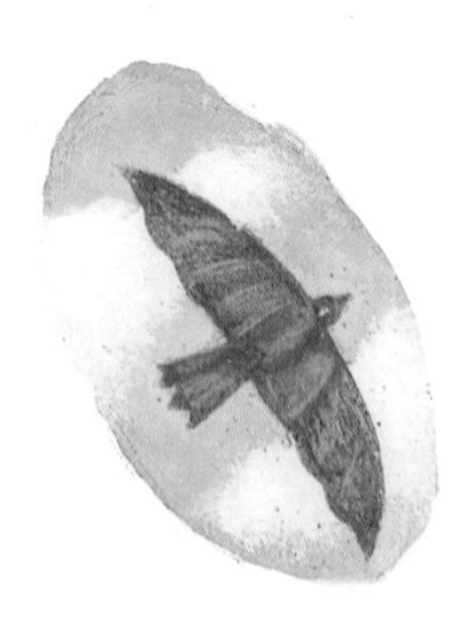

Transcendence is based upon trust. If we trust the spirit world, we surrender our will to the One Will and thus transcend earthly concerns. On the other hand, we experience spiritual defeat when we hold tight to something that is not working. Or if we refuse to let go of controlling another person. But it is not just control of others and of ideas that we surrender. If we do not want a spiritual defeat, we must learn to surrender our human power into the hands of Spirit, of All That Is, of our Source. There is no defeat for our soul.

WHEN YOU DRAW THIS CARD you may be called upon to make a sacrifice.

If the card is UPRIGHT, you work well with the concept of surrender and transcendence. It may be that you need to be more grounded to the earth and its principles. Do not become too lofty and spacey. Keep your feet on the ground and move along the continuum toward the middle.

If the card is REVERSED, you must not accept defeat of your highest principles and ideals. You may be holding on too tight to ideals and principles that are outdated or outmoded and are no longer working for the good of someone you love.

REFLECT on what it is you need to let go of. This surrender is not just letting go but placing your own human will in alignment with the One Will. Act for the common good.

AFFIRM with feeling: "I sanctify my Reiki path with willingness and joy. As above, so below."

TRANSCENDENCE MEDITATION

- Move to a place deep within yourself, for this ceremony will change your life.
- Take an inventory of your qualities, characteristics, and attributes. Think about the effects of the Archetypal Reiki work in your life.
- You find yourself in a grand golden temple. You know that it is the temple of the Great Beaming Light, the temple that you've read about in which the spirit of past Reiki masters and teachers live. You know that this temple resides within your soul.
- You are dressed in a white ceremonial robe. The robe has Reiki symbols embroidered in gold down the front and on the pockets. There is a large golden om on the back of the robe.
- You move into the altar room and before you is a beautiful Archetypal Reiki altar. There are two candelabra on either side of the altar, a beautiful embroidered altar cloth that is the same as the robe you are wearing. In the center of the altar is a large ceremonial silver burning bowl. You know that this is the sacrificial bowl in this temple. You sit at the side of the altar at a writing table. You pick up a quill pen and you write about what in your life you need to sacrifice. It may be the outcome of a certain project. It may be a relationship. It may be your pride, arrogance, fear, ego needs, greed, or any number of qualities, characteristics, and attributes you cannot hold tight to if you wish to progress spiritually.

- When you examine your heart and your soul, you are ready and willing to sacrifice what you've written on the paper. You feel deeply humble and deeply trusting that this ceremony is right for you.
- You carry the paper up the three steps before the altar. You kneel and say your prayer of surrender. Then you stand up, hold the paper to the flame of the candle on your right. As the flame takes hold of the paper, you know that with the flame, you are being purified.
- You drop the burning paper, with your sacrifice on it, into the burning bowl. As the smoke rises from the burning bowl, you feel your spirit rise in transcendence. You feel clear and clean and purified. You give thanks and return to your life, better than you were before.

15. TORII: THE GATEWAY

Be willing to walk a spiritual path. Make preparations for the next part of your spiritual journey. Strengthen yourself physically, emotionally, and/or spiritually. Become willing to trust and move in faith.

The concept of torii is as ancient as Japan itself. The torii is a gate that marks the entrance to the sacred grounds of a Shinto shrine and indicates that the area inside is sacred space. It can be made of all kinds of materials, from unpainted trees to stone or even concrete. The styles of torii vary with the diverse variety of rituals and ideas included in the Shinto shrine worship.

In spiritual terms, when you pass through a door or a gate, you change into spirit form and the gateway protects and shelters your spirit from harm. A gate is a seat of wisdom and signifies new opportunities for spiritual renewal. In Archetypal Reiki work, we use the concept of the torii as an initiation entrance and a signal to ourselves that we must enter an altered state of consciousness in order to perform our ritual graciously.

Within this archetype are two poles, willingness and willfulness. Whenever we do spiritual work, we must prepare our personalities to cross a threshold into another state of consciousness. We must be willing to move into the spirit realm. The will, or willpower, is the executive of the personality. It carries out or executes what we understand to be right or good or true. Willingness means choice, volition. It is based on trust. If we trust, then we surrender. And what we surrender is our willpower. We give our power to God.

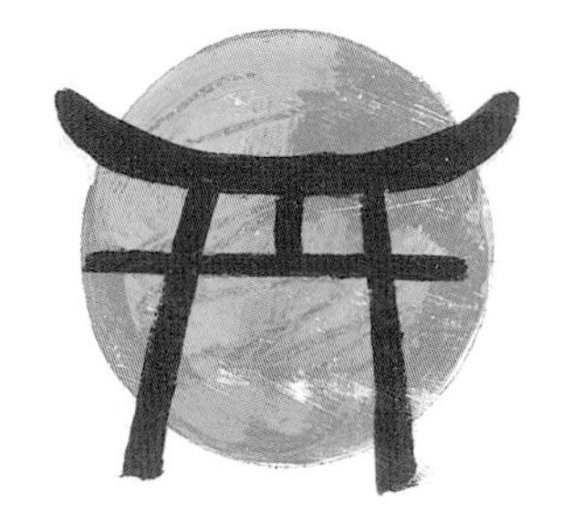

If we attempt to do our spiritual work in an ordinary state of consciousness, we will not be prepared for the changes that come with devotion. To make progress, we must be willing to move into the spiritual realm. We cannot cling stubbornly to old ways and old understandings or refuse to accept new truths. To succeed in our spiritual work, we must not be willful or unreasoningly obstinate.

Spiritual understanding rises up from within through intuition and inspiration. Like any task on the earthly plane, willingness is often gained by loosening our stubborn hold on things and preparing for our journey.

WHEN YOU DRAW THIS CARD in a reading you must make preparations for the next part of your spiritual journey.

If the card is UPRIGHT, your preparations are going well. You have everything you need for the journey to the mountain.

If the card is REVERSED, you still have not prepared yourself for the next lap of your journey. Perhaps you need to work on willingness.

EXERCISE: You need to gather together what you need for your journey. This can be done symbolically or physically. If your journey is to be on the physical level, you might want to search out a spiritual retreat or a spiritually directed tour. These can be found in any of the "new age" or metaphysical magazines. If your work is to be done symbolically, your willingness is indicated when you work with your deck.

AFFIRM with feeling: "As I gather together what I need to prepare for my spiritual journey, I ask for willingness and trust from my spirit masters and guides. Thank you."

TORII MEDITATION

- Go to the place within you where your inner self dwells. Allow this inner self to bask in the light of spiritual understanding, of what you understand to be right and true at this point in time. If, for example, you have been programmed to believe that might makes right (or some other such concept), you now have come to understand that this is an untruth. You must now exercise your will to manifest in the world another idea: the idea that what is right and true will prevail in the material world because it is based on spiritual principles that transcend mere matter.
- You see before you a torii, an entranceway into the spiritual realm. Your knees feel weak, you perspire and you tremble a little. You realize that, once you pass through the entranceway, you will never be the same. You know that you must use your will to move your feet. You are so frightened because you do not know what

you will become. Yet you willingly use the tools that you've learned through your Archetypal Reiki work with the healing cards. You pray, ask for guidance, you meditate and ask for willingness. You feel humble and reverent.

- Something releases deep within you and you know you have achieved the willingness to proceed on your spiritual journey.
- You move through the gateway. You give thanks for the new opportunity.

16. THE WATERFALL: CLEANSING AND CLEARING

Water can dissolve, absolve, wash away, and regenerate. Water represents the cosmos in its entirety. It is the liquid counterpart of light. As rain, it is the inseminating power of the sky god, fertility. As dew, it is benediction and blessing.

Waterfalls are a part of Shinto shrine rituals. It is said that Dr. Usui meditated by the waterfall before he ascended Mount Kuriyama. Waterfalls are brought into being by water falling from a higher place to a lower place, signifying the unity of the Divine and the Human. Because of its great height, the waterfall has the tremendous power of water in motion, symbolizing new creative potential.

In the purification rites of the ancient world, one enters the waterfall naked to show one's vulnerability and openness to the power of God. The pool at the bottom of the waterfall encloses the sacred and is the pool of purification. One stands under the waterfall to show humility and asks to be cleansed of all disease and impurities and re-created pure of heart.

Water itself is undifferentiated, unmanifest, potential energy. Water is the first form of matter and is associated with mother, birth, and the womb of the earth, prima materia. There is a Japanese concept called nagáre. It means the flow of life. Water flows in successive moments of endless renewal. Rivers, lakes, streams, and other bodies of water but especially waterfalls are favored as places of meditation and purification, renewal and re-creation. Water in all its forms is a wonderful metaphor for Life.

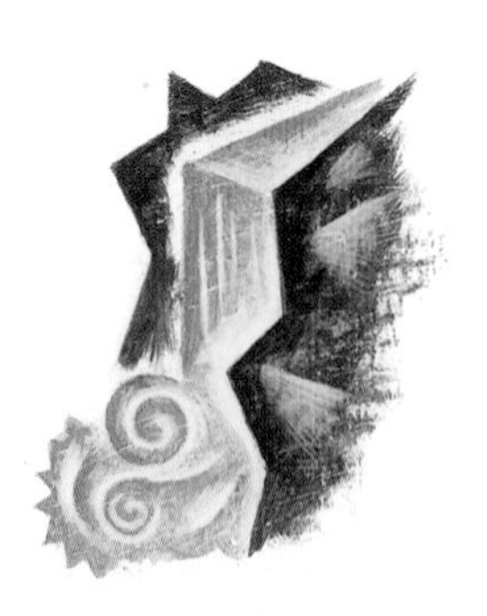

The two opposing forces in this archetype are purification and contamination. When we live at the purification end of the continuum, we tend to perform purification rituals too often, indicating fear and a lack of trust in the Universe. Living at this end might show up in compulsive habits such as showering too often, too vigorously, or obsessively washing your hands. When we notice our habits becoming compulsive, we need to move toward the other end of the continuum, while avoiding contamination.

When we live at the contamination end of the spectrum, we are careless about our health, whether it's physical, emotional, mental, or spiritual health. We adapt to a contaminated world. We must move toward the middle or more toward the purification end if we are to remain healthy.

WHEN YOU DRAW THIS CARD in a reading, know that you are being asked to purify something in your life. Perhaps you are too excessive in one or more of your habits. Perhaps you are neglecting another area of your life that needs cleansing and clearing.

If the card is UPRIGHT, you tend to use purification rituals appropriately and moderately. Try this ritual: Create a prayer of gratitude. Write it on a paper and fold the paper in half. Hang your prayer somewhere special to you and consecrate the area around it.

If the card is REVERSED, you need to do a purification ritual using water. Here is a good one: After making a prayer for something you desire, prepare your bath, using sea salt or some other purifying agent. If desired, place some seashells in the water. As you bathe or shower, symbolically re-create a waterfall or the life-giving waters of some sacred place. Imagine the colors of the rainbow washing through each of your chakras as they open and vibrate with love and energy.

GIVE THANKS when you are finished. Your prayer is already answered.

REFLECT: In ancient times, people stood under the waterfall to feel the power of the water rushing to the earth and to cleanse their hearts and souls. A modern equivalent is standing under the shower, feeling the power of the water cleansing you.

REFLECT ON WATER AS FLOW: Remember the Japanese concept of nagáre, which means to flow with each moment of your life, letting go of each past moment. In the succession of water, of now moments, we recognize that all things will come to pass in God's time.

AFFIRM with feeling: "As I allow the waterfall to cover my head and body, so I allow God to cover my entire being with love and abundance. I live in gratitude for my blessings."

WATERFALL MEDITATION

- You have moved through the torii into sacred space. You feel, though, that you are contaminated with the world's energy. The impurities and corruption of the external world nag at you. You feel as if you have a disease. Your skin is not clear. Your eyes are not clear. And you do not hear acutely. You have picked up the cares of the world and have not yet been purified.
- You see before you a sparkling waterfall cascading down the Cosmic Mountain.
- The waterfall contains the full spectrum, all the colors of the rainbow within its waters.
- You feel that some of your chakras have become blocked. You drop your daily clothes and you step naked into the colored waterfall.
- As you stand there with the warm, cleansing waters rushing over your body, you feel your mind, heart, and soul also being purified. Your thoughts turn to spiritual matters. You feel love in your heart and your soul rises up to meet the Source.
- When you feel the spiritual energy returning to your being, you step out of the rushing waterfall and into the warm, white robe of Archetypal Reiki. You know that you will forever remember the concept of nagáre and of living life in successive now moments. You drink a glass of pure, clear water and feel it cleanse your soul as you return to your life.

17. DRAGON'S BREATH: SPIRITUAL INITIATION

Use the dragon as a spirit guide and its breath will strengthen your ki. Try saying this: With the dragon's breath, I blow power into my soul.

The dragon is a powerful symbol that represents life force and great potency. This is the time to step into your power. Dragons also guard treasure. The treasure that your dragon guards may be your precious Higher Self.

In ancient times it was thought that, hidden in a cave guarded by a dragon, lay a horde of gold and jewels. This symbolism commonly represents the spiritual wisdom buried in the unconscious. The winged dragon is a powerful symbol of transcendence and can mean ascension to spiritual and mystical heights. The dragon's breath is like the fire of purification. A dragon's breath ceremony is part of the Reiki tradition.

In Christianity and in the Shinto religion there is also a tradition of purification by fire. Here we use the fire of the dragon's breath to purify, to symbolize power and the passion to heal ourselves and our planet.

Within this archetype are the two poles of alignment and misalignment. In Archetypal Reiki work, alignment simply means to be in tune with Reiki energy, lined up.

At the other end of the continuum is misalignment, where a person is not in tune with the spiritual healing energy that is all around us. When we move toward the middle of this archetype, we utilize the symbology of the dragon's breath to align ourselves with spiritual energy in all forms.

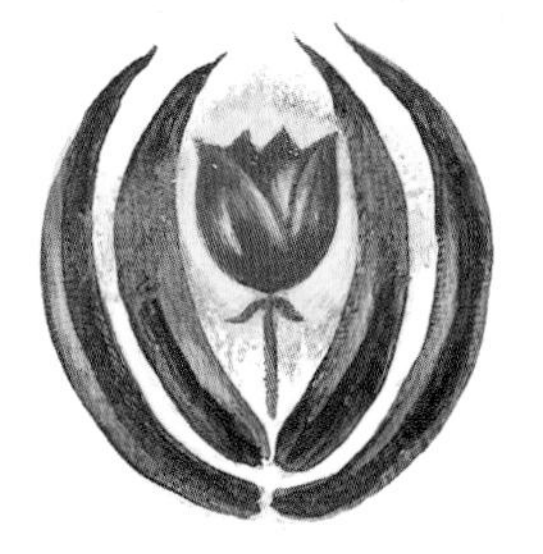

WHEN YOU DRAW THIS CARD it is a signal to step into your own power, the power of the dragon. Think of the dragon as a powerful ally that can help you to build up and contain your power. Use the dragon as a spirit guide and its breath will strengthen your ki.

If the card is UPRIGHT, you are in tune with the spiritual energy all around you. You may, however, be too consciously aware of yourself. To be self-conscious is to ignore spirit-consciousness.

If the card is REVERSED, you are asked to tune yourself to the spiritual energy of the Dragon's Breath card work.

One reason we may be out of alignment with spiritual energy is because we restrict our breathing by holding the belly muscles too tight. We must learn to soften the belly muscles.

TRY THIS EXERCISE DAILY: Lie down on your back. Rest your arms at your sides and bend your knees so that your feet are flat on the floor. As you inhale, fill your belly with air and gently arch the small of your back. As you exhale, flatten the small of your back. Keep it slow and gentle.

AFFIRM with feeling: "I empower myself with the Breath of the Dragon."

DRAGON'S BREATH MEDITATION

- You are in a misty, foggy place with lots of stone around. It is an ancient place. You feel the power of this place and know you are here for an important reason. You are here to do the work of the dragon.
- You see a wonderful, large, old tree with hanging branches. In its shade is a carved stone bench. You sit on the bench and look all around you. A single golden flower seems to call you. You stare at it, and in its center you see emerging a beautiful gold and green dragon. Fire comes out of the dragon's nostrils, but it is not a fire that consumes. It is the fire of purification. You ask the dragon if it is here to help you. It tells you through mental telepathy that, yes, it is here to help you as long as you need its fire power and energy.
- The dragon indicates that you are to climb on its back and hold on to the spikes on its neck. You comply, though you are afraid. You find that the spikes do not hurt, for they are covered in soft leather. As the dragon moves over the earth and through the air, you find you are enjoying the power and freedom the ride gives you. You feel you are being infused with the power of the dragon. You find that, as you breathe, your exhalations resemble the dragon's breath, for the two of you have become one.
- You know that you have now stepped into your own spiritual power, with the help of the spirit world. You thank God.

18. THE CAVE: STRUGGLE WITH EGO

Go within yourself, into your deep unconscious. Willingly enter the dark places within yourself and be utterly honest. Bring these parts of yourself into the light where you can see them clearly.

In ancient cultures the cave was a sacred place of initiation, representing the home of the spirits who ruled the preliterate imagination. The cave is a cosmic center as well as the feminine yin principle, internal and hidden, within the mountain. The cave is a womb, warm, dark, and comforting. It represents the unconscious or the entrance to the underworld. The cave symbolizes the place of spiritual retreat in which there must be a union of ego and soul and a meeting of the Divine and the human.

There is ancient wisdom stored in the caves of the unconscious, but to get to it we must undergo a process of initiation, entering the secret cave by a labyrinth or dangerous passage. Passing through the cave, like moving through the torii, represents a change of state, a change in consciousness.

The cave in Archetypal Reiki work symbolizes a place of entry, a place deep in the womb of the earth. A place where we descend into the darkness. In the darkness, we meet our Shadow, the unaccepted part of our personality. The struggle between our Higher Self and our Shadow takes place in the cave. It is here we merge ego and soul to create a new synergy that works for our spiritual growth. Both the shadow of the ego and the light of our soul must be embraced and balanced for us to be healthy.

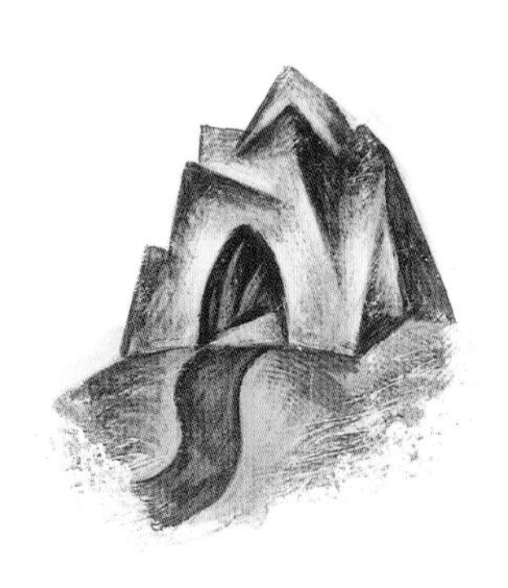

Within this archetype are the two opposite polarities, humility and ego-control. If we live at the humility end of the continuum, we may become a doormat for those who need to walk over others, to take advantage of good-heartedness. We must stand our ground in matters that are important to us, for if we have too much humility too much of the time, we will be in trouble. We must allow ego to function in a healthy manner. We must set limits on the behavior of others.

On the other end of the continuum, if we have too much ego-control, we become rigid and harsh to ourselves and to others. If we have too much ego-control, it means that we are closed to anything or anyone we cannot understand with the rational mind.

WHEN YOU DRAW THIS CARD it is a signal for you to go within yourself, into your deep unconscious. You are being asked to willingly enter the dark places within yourself and be utterly honest. Bring these parts of yourself into the light where you can see them.

If the card is UPRIGHT, you tend to have spiritual humility. You may need to watch that other people don't take advantage of your good heart—or of your fear.

If the card is REVERSED, your tendency is toward ego-control. You must watch that your need to control others does not harm you or them. You also must watch your tendency to put controls on yourself that are too tight for your own good. Lighten up.

EXERCISE: Write about three things that most block your spiritual progress. If your ego gets in the way, describe what you mean by "ego." If you are distracted by earthly concerns, describe what distracts you and how you become distracted. If you appear to be "lazy," describe what that is and how it feels and how it blocks your progress.

AFFIRM with feeling: "As I enter the cave of my deepest self, may I be willing to wrestle with my darkness, [name the area of most concern to you], so that I may be spiritually enlightened and move up the mountain."

CAVE MEDITATION

- You are on the last leg of the long journey to your Higher Self. The external world has been holding you hostage for many years now. You have taken steps to shed this burden. You have entered sacred space through the torii. You have stood beneath the magic waterfall and been purified. You have been initiated with the dragon's breath into a spiritual life. Still, something oppresses you and burdens your heart and soul. When you felt the breath of the dragon and rode on its back, you felt the pull of power. And it got to you. It entered your psyche in a place where ego lives. Sure enough! Despite all your precautions, you have found yourself in a power struggle with another person or even with yourself. You know that your shadow-ego is at work again.

- You journey to the holy mountain. At its base you find a labyrinth that looks dangerous. There are many curves in it, many passages dark with underbrush where no sun shines. You see no other way to enter the cave that you intuitively know is at the end of the labyrinth.
- You have prepared yourself well. You have eaten good, raw, unpreserved food. You have exercised your body until it is fit and strong. You have prayed long and hard in your private temple. You have dressed yourself in the ceremonial robes fit for such an undertaking.
- You shed your clothes and anoint yourself with oil and with the holy red earth of the mountain base. You fast and meditate for two days and three nights. On the morning of the third day, your inner guidance tells you that you are ready. You invoke your spirit guides and the Reiki masters to help you as you enter the labyrinth.
- For ten days you travel through the dark and dangerous labyrinth, seeking the cave where you must do your work. You arrive finally at the exit and there before you is the cave where your Higher Self must integrate both ego and soul. Where the battle for your soul takes place.
- Deep in the cave you go, your guides at your side. There is your ego, your intellect with its strident I want! I need! Gimme! Gimme now! And its logical conclusions that don't make intuitive sense at all. The ego wrestles for control with your poetic soul. Your intuition doesn't make sense to your ego either. There must be a compromise! The ego gets a headlock on the soul, and back and forth they go, battling for your very life.
- The shadows move on the wall of the cave. Light and dark, light and dark. Finally, ego and soul embrace as they say, "Good job! Well done! I see your point!"
- Finally they dance the dance of life. Together.
- And it is over! You have won your soul! Rejoice and give thanks!

19. THE SACRED TREE: DEVOTION TO THE SACRED

The sacred tree gives life to the world. Meditate and reflect upon your relationship to the trees around you. Remember, trees symbolize human beings.

The tree—nourishing, protecting, sheltering, and supporting—symbolizes feminine, or yin, energy. Trees with pairs of intertwining boughs signify the pairs of opposites, yin and yang. With its branches reaching to the sky and feeding on the sun and its roots planted deep in the earth, the sacred tree forms a bridge between the heavenly realm of God and the earthly realm of humans. The tree represents diversity in unity with its many branches. A tree is basically a symbol of the Great Awakening.

Japanese Shinto shrines are surrounded by a grove of trees. Sometimes a special tree or rock is selected within the forest and the deities are asked to enter and make their home there. The bough of the tree can be used as an offering during a spiritual ceremony, since it is the branching of the tree that is the embodiment of dynamic life.

In Archetypal Reiki work, the tree is used to symbolize differentiation on the earth plane, and as a symbol of the undying spirit of humankind.

Within this archetype are the two poles of reverence and profanity. To revere something means to regard it with devotion and awe. If we revere common objects too much, we forget our Source. Thus we cannot live at this end of the continuum for long.

On the other hand, we must not be blasphemous or sacrilegious. If we live at this end, we become too secular and uninterested in things sacred. We must move toward the middle in our daily affairs.

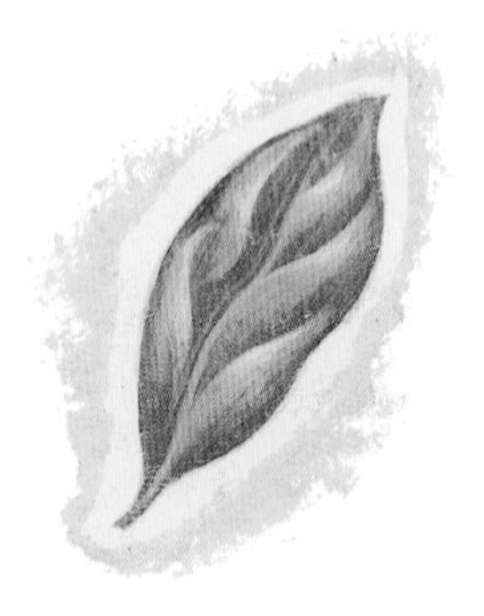

WHEN YOU DRAW THIS CARD you are to meditate and reflect upon the trees around you.

If the card is UPRIGHT, you have great reverence for Nature and the things of Nature. You may need to build up your reverence for human beings.

If the card is REVERSED, you need to work on becoming more reverent toward things sacred and also reverent for things of the earth.

EXERCISE: Go to a neighboring tree. Sit under this tree and tune in to its energy and its wisdom. Listen carefully for the voice of the tree. It may match your own inner voice. Also listen for the voice of a neighboring human.

AFFIRM with feeling: "As I align my human energy with the tree energy, may I walk in beauty upon the earth and build reverence for my environment."

SACRED TREE MEDITATION

- You are deep in the forest. Shadows fall among the trees and into the shrubbery of the forest.
- You move on a path that you have found. It is not the main path, but a side opening into the world of trees and forest animals.
- While on your path, you feel a different kind of energy. You recognize after a while that it is the energy of the trees you are feeling. You stop for a while and sit on a fallen log, listening. The tree itself can be an oracle.
- As you tune to the energy, you notice that the energy of one particular tree calls to you. Your eye lights upon this tree. You move toward it, put your arms around it, and listen for its heartbeat. Sure enough, you feel the heartbeat and your own heart resonates with the energy of this tree. As you stand there fully attuned now, you notice that your feet feel deeply planted in the earth. You feel you have grown roots, and your roots take nourishment from the earth. You seek the life-giving water under the ground. You are rooted and you don't want to move. As you look around, you find that you seem to have grown many arms. You look at them and they are thicker where they are connected to your body and thinner where they branch out into tiny twigs that hold your . . . leaves! For you have become a tree!
- You feel delighted with this transformation and you remain for many years, happily absorbing food, drink, light, and love from your environment. Then one day you notice that you have returned to human form, and you know that you will never again be indifferent to trees, after having lived as one for many years.
- Give thanks for this experience.

20. THE MOUNTAIN: SPIRITUAL ATTAINMENT

You are moving to a higher level of spirituality. Strive for the highest possible level of spiritual development.

In Japan, as elsewhere, mountains are sacred places. They are a meeting place of heaven and earth, symbolizing the masculine, or yang, principle, external and visible.

The mountain represents constancy, firmness, stillness, and, on a more concrete level, an attainable goal or opportunity. We climb mountains to gain purity and protection against ill fortune. The mountaintop represents the state of full consciousness. After we have done the work of the cave, we can climb our mountain to a higher state of consciousness and gain wisdom.

The mountain is a cosmic center. We can identify our own spine with the mountain's central axis, and in so doing we become cosmic. Our bodies rotate around their axial points as the world revolves around its center.

In Archetypal Reiki work, the mountain is a passage from one plane to a higher one where we can communicate more fully with God.

Within the mountain archetype are the two opposing forces of wisdom and absurdity. Wisdom is a deep, global understanding of what is true, right, or lasting. Wisdom includes good judgment. It is characteristic of wisdom not to do desperate things. Wisdom itself is balance. It is when we think we are all-wise and all-perfect that we become insufferable. It is when we think we "know it all" that our wisdom deserts us and we must move away from the extreme.

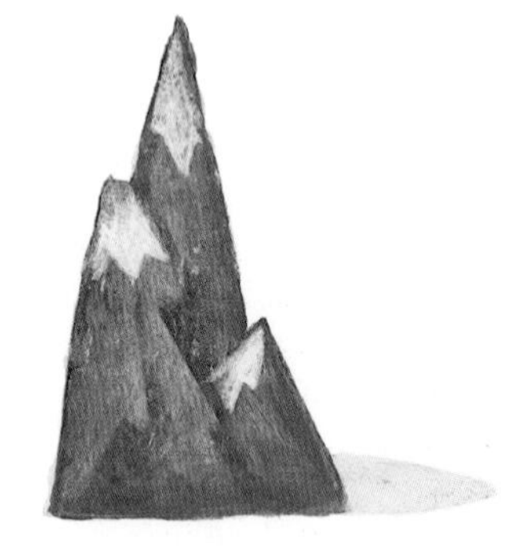

When we accept the philosophical position that life is an absurd joke, nothing means much to us and we lose all sense of values. It often appears that life is absurd and sometimes it truly is, but we must move toward the middle of the continuum to appreciate life and its vicissitudes. We also must learn to laugh at the absurdity of life and of ourselves. Laughter is not considered to be a spiritual virtue, but it should be. Think about how often you truly, genuinely laugh.

WHEN YOU DRAW THIS CARD in a reading know that you are moving to a higher level of spirituality. In reality, there is no "higher" or "lower" level of development. All that is certain is that we draw our soul out into the Light with spiritual growth. What we think of as "higher" is really a drawing out of our soul.

When the card is UPRIGHT, you are on the right path. Do a ritual of gratitude for all you've been given and meditate on your mountain for the next week.

When the card is REVERSED, you are in for a new death (transformation)—meaning that after a symbolic death comes the rebirth. Something new is coming.

EXERCISE: Do the mountain meditation slowly every day for the next week and journal your experience. When you do the meditation, pretend your spine is the axis of the Cosmic Mountain. Be the mountain.

AFFIRM with feeling: "As I ascend my spiritual mountain in search of wisdom, the journey becomes more lonely. I accept this and I thank my god and my spirit guides for the journey."

MOUNTAIN MEDITATION

- You have been traveling your path for many years, perhaps many lifetimes. You are nearing a plateau along your journey to wholeness and wisdom. You have made peace with the external world at this point in time. You feel ready to go farther.
- As you walk along the path that has chosen you, you slip on loose rock and find yourself flat on the ground. No, you realize that you are the ground. You are flat and spread out as far as you can see. People walk on your surface, but you don't mind. That's your purpose in life: to ground spiritual travelers to the earth of which they are a part.
- As you reflect on your purpose in life, you notice that you have grown. You have seemed to become thicker all over and higher than you could imagine. In your core of rock there seems to be a stable point, a center stillness. It is your axis, you realize.
- Wonderful green trees seem to have sprouted all over your face. Someone has carefully carved roads into your sides, and you don't mind at all. Spiritual seekers seem

to be compelled to climb your face and to feel the winds of change at your head. Your head is up very high, often in the clouds. The breath of God blows all around your head and you are at peace. You have been here for eons. You have grown organically, out of the earth's activity and out of the earth's center. You are part of the earth and yet also part of those who seek transcendence. It is enough. You are at peace.

21. JINJA SHINTO: THE SHRINE OF THE SOUL

Create a ritual, if you do not already have one, in which you contact the Spirit and your own Higher Self on a daily basis.

Jinja shrine is a Shinto shrine devoted to the worship of kami. There is no literal translation for the word *kami*; it means something like the divine spark in everything in the Universe, the god within. Stuart Picken, a scholar who has studied and written about Shinto practices, describes kami as "anything that can inspire a sense of wonder and awe in the beholder, in a way that testifies to the divinity of its origin or being." In Archetypal Reiki work, the things that fit Picken's description are called Spirit or Source or God. From this Source we ask for protection from negative influences or assistance with something in our daily life. It is here we take refuge and seek shelter from the storms and stress of life. We are on the long journey of the soul into Light.

We define the shrine of the soul as any sacred place or space that is designated by an individual for his or her own devotion. The shrine of the soul can be an open space, a building in which sacred space is set aside, or any altar, natural or man-made. Or the shrine of the soul can be a place deep within a person, which is consecrated as a sacred place within.

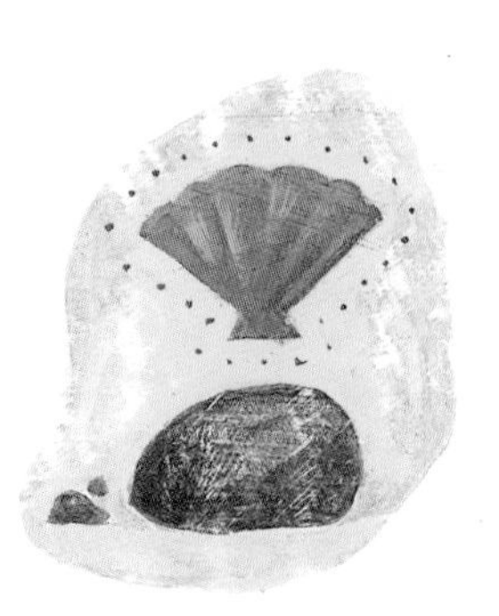

Within this archetype are two polarities, commitment and refusal. We are asked to live at the commitment end of this spectrum. Commitment means a trust. We trust that to which we are committed. When we commit to an idea or a person or to God, we are pledging or promising our fidelity to this cause. A commitment is not to be taken lightly. Not only must we keep our promise, but we must be certain that we're committed to the path that is for our soul's highest purpose. To be sure of this requires frequent examination of our deeper motives.

We are asked to commit to the

path of spiritual growth, of empowerment. We must not refuse to see the signs and signals of a need for better spiritual practices. If we live at the refusal end of the archetype, we stay in the world of materiality and refuse to grow spiritually.

WHEN YOU DRAW THIS CARD in a reading you are asked to create a ritual.

If the card is UPRIGHT, you may already have an excellent shrine for your soul and a deep commitment to your spiritual path. Think about daily contact with the Source.

If the card is REVERSED, you may be refusing to commit to a path you know you are already on. After doing the shrine of the soul meditation, change your altar space around to include something that comes up for you during this next week. You will be guided to something that serves your soul's highest purpose.

AFFIRM with feeling: "I do not worship my own individual soul. I honor, revere, and worship the divine spark within myself, other people, and the natural world around me. May the spark of divinity burn brightly within my soul and lead me to my highest purpose."

JINJA SHRINE MEDITATION

- You are on a path that winds through a deep woods. You move along quite contentedly, but you know that you still seek something more. You affirm to yourself that you will find what you seek, and you will know it when you find it, very soon. You move through some dense, heavy forest now, and suddenly, you find yourself in a clearing. Before you is a huge white domelike temple. You approach this building with awe, wondering what lives inside. The temple is surrounded by small spires that look like white lace. You can almost see the energetic vibrations. You can feel the presence of mystical beings.
- You enter the front door of the temple and find yourself surrounded by a white mist. You are not frightened, but you are certain that you must move through the mist to find what you seek.
- You come to a quiet, small place, and you know you have found what you've been seeking. In this small, quiet place is a brilliant white light. The light has no form, but you recognize its brilliance and energy as the light of your own soul. You have come to the shrine of your soul. The place where your soul lives and you rejoice as you are reunited with your personal soul. You and your soul dance in celebration. You give thanks.

22. ROOT CHAKRA: PHYSICAL NEEDS

Is something amiss in your physical or work or money life? Remember: You have an inborn right to basic safety and security in life.

The Path of Manifestation. The first three chakras—the root, the abdomen, and the stomach—form a downward current that, according to Anodea Judith, a leading authority on the integration of chakras and therapeutic issues, is called the Path of Manifestation. This is how we take something abstract and make it concrete in the external world. We turn spirit into matter.

The root chakra, located at the base of the spinal cord, is considered part of the "lower chakra" system, that which ties us to the earth. This chakra is the basic foundation of our physical life, bringing us safety, security, and a sense of home and family as well as our work life. The ways in which we manifest our reality and live in the present moment are root chakra work.

With this chakra, we are given the right to Be, to Exist. Its color is blood red.

Within this archetype are two opposing forces, high energy and lassitude. With good physical, mental, emotional, and spiritual health comes high physical energy. Physical energy is necessary for our well-being. However, too much activity produces hyperactivity. When this condition arises we cannot sit still, much less meditate. Our minds are continually racing. We must move over to the middle of the archetype.

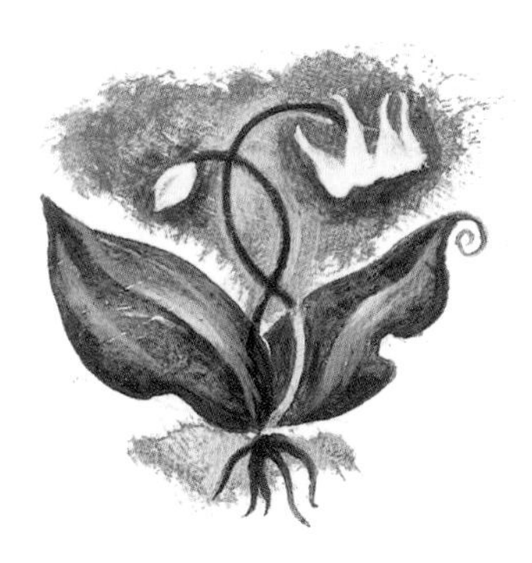

Lassitude occurs when our physical energy is debilitated. This can happen with too much stress, too little solitude, or when we are physically sick. We don't need to wait until we feel weak or exhausted to relax and re-create ourselves. We need to care for ourselves before we get into this condition. We need to move toward balance.

WHEN YOU DRAW THIS CARD in your reading you are advised that something may be amiss. In which area of your life do you feel the pull?

When the card is UPRIGHT, you need more grounding to the earth plane on a daily basis. You often walk around with your "head in the clouds." (See Card No. 11, Grounding and Balance.)

When this card is REVERSED, you are too laid-back. This often means that you are not involved or caring or even that you are depressed. You need to be energized at the physical level. Wear a lot of red and burn red candles as you ask for help in this area.

EXERCISE: Make a chart of where you are offbalance in your physical life. The chart could include body (diet, rest, exercise, bathroom habits, using your senses daily to experience the world); finances (work you like, adequate income—manageable or no debts—money allocated for "fun," money allocated for others, if possible); work life (work you enjoy or plans to change work situation); car (reliable transportation); even plans for further education.

AFFIRM with feeling: "I live in an abundant universe. I have a right to share in the abundance of God's physical world. I am rich."

ROOT CHAKRA MEDITATION

- You are lying in a bed in a warm, comfortable, softly lit room. You hear soul-stirring music, lullaby music. The smell of fresh flowers fills the room.
- An angel comes to your bedside and places a tiny, newborn babe in your arms. The angel tells you that you have just given birth to your Divine Child.
- You gaze at the face of the child and you know it is true. You have just given birth to yourself. You are overjoyed and thrilled. Your soul is deeply moved. Your heart sings.
- You rock the child and suckle the little one at your breast. As the child feeds from your body, you tell this child that you are glad she was born. You have waited a very long time for this miraculous birth, the birth of yourself into the world. You tell the child that you love her unconditionally and that you will always protect her.
- You communicate to the child that when she cries in the night, you will hear. You will listen to the soft murmuring of her soul and the pain of her heart. The child's joy will be your joy. You will run through lovely meadows with this child, seeking

together the peace and comfort that comes with pure love. You will never abandon her but will cherish her always in your heart.

- When you finish nursing your Divine Child, tell her that she will always live inside of you, where it is forever safe and secure. And then return to your life and keep your promises.

23. ABDOMINAL CHAKRA: CREATION AND SEXUALITY

Examine your sexuality and look for ways you could be more satisfied sexually. Examine your creativity and look for ways you might be more satisfied creatively.

The abdominal chakra, also called the spleen chakra or sacral chakra, is located at the womb level and is a part of the "lower chakra" system, that which connects us to the earth. This chakra is connected to the underground river of creativity.

The abdominal chakra is sometimes called the hara. This is where the Samurai committed hara-kiri in old Japan, piercing the most vulnerable place in themselves in honor of an ideal.

This is the place of reproduction and creativity, which come from the same source. It is the watery place where emotions are produced and stored. The work of this chakra is about how we relate to people and how we seek validation. The work of this chakra is to let go of any guilt we feel and to stay connected to ourselves and to others. And to our own creativity.

This chakra gives us the right to feel. It is bright orange.

Within this archetype are the two opposite characteristics of creation and destruction. We are all creative. Whether we create a picture, a piece of music, a sculpture, or our own life, we are cocreators with God. Our passion for life, for our children, and for the products of our creativity lives in this chakra. At the creative end of the continuum, be certain you are creating what you want to create and what is for your soul's highest purpose.

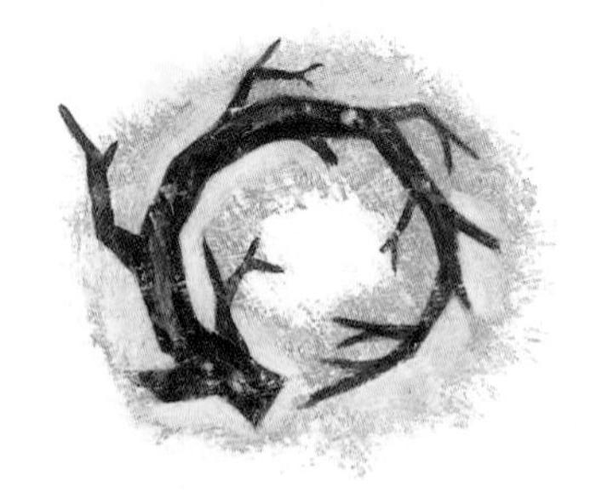

At the other end of the continuum lies disaster. We cannot live with destruction, although at times we need to tear something down and begin again. This is true of ideas, feelings, and the products of our dreams. It takes much more time and energy to create than it does to destroy, yet often we kill the very thing we love the most. Move to the middle or the other end of the continuum.

WHEN YOU DRAW THIS CARD in a reading you are being asked to examine your sexuality.

If the card is UPRIGHT, you are in touch with both your sexuality and your creativity. You know they come from the same source. You are not upset when, as so often happens, one is more dormant and the other more dominant. The scales will change.

If the card is REVERSED, you need to be more in touch with yourself. You need to know yourself better. Examine your needs and how you fill them.

EXERCISE: Every day, write down three feelings about your sexuality. Then write three feelings about your creativity. After a week, see if there's a discernible pattern.

Wear orange and burn an orange candle as you ask for help in releasing your stored emotions through your creativity or your sexuality.

AFFIRM with feeling: "My spleen chakra releases all stored emotions and I am free to express myself in constructive and productive ways."

ABDOMINAL CHAKRA MEDITATION

- At this time in your life, your creativity seems to be blocked. Your passion seems to have spent itself. You feel dull and disinterested.
- One night, in your sleep, your creative spirit guides come to you and tell you that, if you are willing, they will take you on a journey to find your sexuality and/or your creativity. They will help you to find a way to tap into your passion once again.
- You are in a beautiful Gothic cathedral. You have been there for some time, lighting candles and deep in prayer. You move out of the main body of the cathedral and to the courtyard, where you find a warm rainbow fountain. You sit on the bench in front of the fountain and meditate. You look deep into the center of the rainbow fountain and you find yourself drawn into the water right in the center. You move down, down, down to the bottom of the fountain. Into the earth deep beneath the fountain.
- Deep in the earth you find a river. An underground river of creativity. Deep in the river, you see the faces and you hear the voices of those who have gone before you

in creativity. All of the great writers, painters, sculptors, composers, and other creative people throughout the ages.

- You know that you have come upon the river of the collective unconscious that flows over all of us. You spend many years at this river, moving up and down, in and out of this place. It is a magic place of renewal. It is a mystical place of re-creation.
- When you return to the world, you carry with you gifts from the river. You carry with you gifts from the creative ones who have gone before you. You are one with all, as the river is one with its Source.

24. SOLAR PLEXUS CHAKRA: ACTION IN THE WORLD

Look at the ways you handle personal power. You may be exerting undue influence over other people, not allowing them to feel their own power. Be sure you act in your own best interests as well as those of others.

The solar plexus chakra is located at the stomach level. It is the last of the earthbound chakras. As the seat of personal identity, the solar plexus provides the empowerment to act upon our beliefs and values. Thinking, categorizing, planning, organizing, and discriminating are the work of the power center. The solar plexus chakra shows us how we can be more effective in our lives and how we can link the soul with the ego. It connects us with our firepower of action in the world, in which there is no shame.

With this chakra we have the right to act. The color for the stomach chakra is sunshine yellow.

Within this archetype are the two opposite characteristics of empowerment and disempowerment. At the empowerment end of the continuum, we feel an extraordinary sense of our own internal power. When we are at this end of the continuum, we must be sure that we are not feeling or acting out "power over" another in our sense of self.

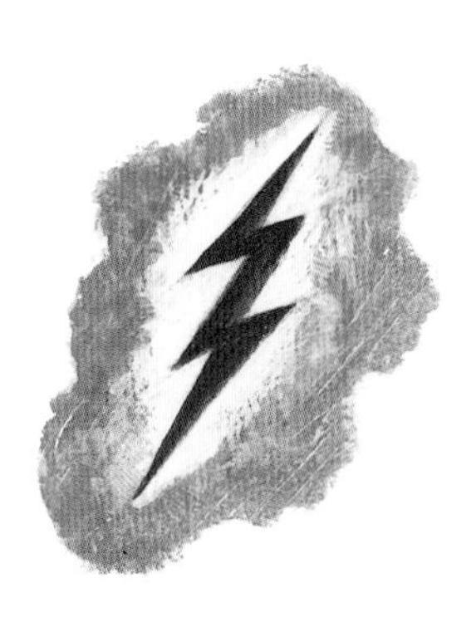

The stomach chakra offers us a sense of our own identity, of who we are, which includes our feelings about ourselves and who we are in the world around us. It is the seat of self-esteem, self-confidence, and self-worth.

When we feel totally disempowered, we have no ability to make a plan, carry it out, and feel good about ourselves. Disempowerment, in fact, results in soul loss, in holes in our soul. We have to be careful when we are at this end of the spectrum that we do not allow others to have power over us either. If others have too much unwarranted power over us, we feel disempowered, weak, and helpless. We need our power inside, where we can draw upon it.

WHEN YOU DRAW THIS CARD you are advised to look at the ways you handle personal power.

When the card is UPRIGHT, you use your personal power well, neither controlling nor allowing yourself to be controlled.

When the card is REVERSED, you may not feel your own power nor your own ability to do things for yourself. You may be too dependent on others to think for you or to act for you.

EXERCISE: Every day, take deep stomach breaths and ask for your personal empowerment.

AFFIRM with feeling: "As I breathe, I bring power into my solar plexus. I become more empowered daily through the breath of God."

SOLAR PLEXUS CHAKRA MEDITATION

- Be with your inner self now. You are in a clearing in the woods. You have been here, doing rituals, for days, perhaps weeks. You need to feel your own power. The fire is burning brightly. The fire is burning hot. The fire is here.
- Circle the fire.
- Feel the power of the fire.
- Dance the dance of the fire.
- Dance away from the heat of the fire.
- You are once more a child of the forest. The smell of burning wood comforts you. See the flames, living orange-red flames in the night. The snapping, popping sounds fall upon the hard gray ground at your feet. Dance the dance of power.
- As you do this ritual before the fire, you become a flame. A flame that burns through all your fears, all your sorrow, all your pain. You feel the flame burning through your stomach to your soul. You are empowered by the flame.
- Whenever you feel finished, return to the external world you know, carrying the flame with you.

25. THE HEART CHAKRA: THE MEDIATOR

Examine your feelings, thoughts, and especially your actions concerning love in your life. To be sure you get enough love, you must be willing to love in return.

There is only one chakra in the middle of the chakra system. This is the heart chakra. For the Path of Manifestation to come into existence, we must turn to this chakra.

The heart chakra is in the middle of the body, at the heart level. It handles all kinds of love: self-love, erotic love, filial love, love of others, and universal love. Life in this center deals with the ways in which we give and receive love.

Work with the heart chakra gives us the right to love and be loved. The color of the heart chakra is emerald green.

Within this archetype are two opposing forces, love and indifference. We must begin with self-love. Without a strong sense of self, our love will be at the unconscious merging stage of infancy. Once we love ourselves, we can love others. Universal love is the ability to look beyond the human personality to the soul of the person and to love that soul. However, at the human personality level, people are not always good, kind, and sweet. Often we need to set limits on another's behavior and not express our love at certain points in time in order to allow that person to act in a manner appropriate, realistic, and kind.

The opposite of love is indifference. When we cease loving someone, we become indifferent to them. We don't care. Indifference is a state close to cruelty. To neglect someone is abusive, and indifference is a form of neglect.

On the other hand, when we lose love in our lives, we enter a period of grief. Grief is a reaction to the loss of love. If we lose love, we lose all. We can lose love in many ways: through abuse, neglect, or a closing of our heart-space. To keep love in our lives, we must pay attention and cherish that which we love and not become indifferent to that love which graces our lives.

WHEN YOU DRAW THIS CARD you must examine your heart.

When the card is UPRIGHT, you may be getting too much love in your life. This means that someone is smothering you or trying to control you with love.

When the card is REVERSED, you may not be getting enough love in your life. You may be trying to protect yourself from being hurt by not opening your heart to others. Look at your love relationship with God first and then your Higher Self and your love will spill out into your world.

EXERCISE: Burn a green candle and wear something green every day for one week as you ask for healing in the area of love in your life. Remember that giving and receiving love are the same thing.

AFFIRM with feeling: "There is always enough love to go around in this world. All love comes from God. I love completely and surely."

HEART CHAKRA MEDITATION

- Lie down for this meditation, with knees bent and feet flat on the floor.
- Relax your body. Relax your mind. Remember that love is a feeling of expansion. Go to that place deep within the center of yourself.
- Ask your spirit guides to help you love more deeply and more strongly. Love is giving and receiving, an exchange of energy. There is no sorrow in your heart. There is only love.
- Now, breathe deeply from the abdomen. Take three deep, belly breaths. As you inhale, reach out with your arms and receive love. Breathe in the love of God, of others, and of yourself.
- As you exhale, reach your arms forward and give love. Breathe out the love of God, of others, and of yourself.
- Do this for fifteen minutes.
- When you return to this time and place, return with the feeling of love in your heart, and each time you exhale, breathe out love. Breathe.

26. THE THROAT CHAKRA: COMMUNICATION WITH THE DIVINE

The throat chakra mediates our ability to speak and to hear the truth. It is a divine gift. Be certain that you say what you mean and you mean what you say.

The three upper chakras—the throat, the inner eye, and the crown—lie along the Path of Liberation. On this path, we take something that is bound to a form and gradually free it to encompass greater scope and abstraction. We turn matter into spirit.

With the throat chakra we enter the realm of spiritual development and spiritual empowerment. The throat chakra is located in the neck, at the throat level. This is the chakra that gives us voice. The throat portrays wisdom and communication. It is the center of higher-level creativity, in which we become cocreators with our Source. It also enables us to listen and to hear more clearly the voice of our inner guidance as well as the voices of those around us. It helps us to hear the voice of the divine in the voices of others.

This is the chakra that gives us the right to speak and hear the Truth. Its color is sky blue.

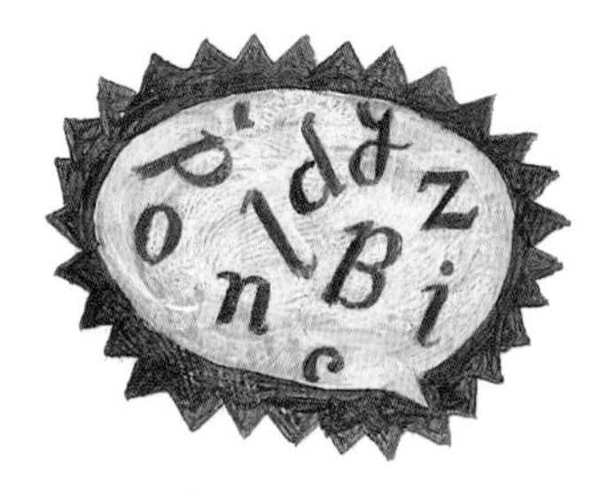

Within this archetype are two opposite characteristics, communication and deafness. To communicate means to make known. To commune with others is an act of sharing ourselves, who we are. To communicate with the Divine means to give and receive, as in prayer and meditation, at the level of Spirit. To communicate with the Divine in ourselves or in other people means to be with or speak with at the soul level.

We communicate in many different ways, at different levels of being. One of the ways we communicate is with our voice. We sing, we chant, we tell stories. We make sounds. Sounds are vibrations, and vibrations are healing. It is said that the first sound God made when the world was created was "om". Sounds become symbols, and through the symbolic world we communicate at ever-higher levels. Through the throat chakra, using our will, we consciously create ourselves out of the God-fabric we are given.

When we do not communicate, we become mute. Do not allow muteness to take over your soul. Use your voice to communicate your soul. And listen with your heart.

WHEN YOU DRAW THIS CARD you need to be certain that you say what you mean and mean what you say. Look at the ways in which you communicate with yourself first and then with others.

If the card is UPRIGHT, you are being emotionally honest and direct. You are being clear and direct with yourself and with others.

If the card is REVERSED, you may not stand behind what you say. You may say things you don't mean. Or you mean things you don't say.

EXERCISE: For the next week, mean what you say and say what you mean. Say whatever needs to be said that you haven't yet expressed. Wear the color blue for the next week and burn a blue candle every day as you ask for help in this area.

AFFIRM with feeling: "I am clear, honest, and direct in my communications with myself and with those around me. I hear the voice of God in the voice of a loved one."

THROAT CHAKRA MEDITATION

- Go to that place deep within yourself that is private, sacred, and safe. In that place, think about and feel the presence of God.
- Now, begin to chant the sound "om". Chant that sound and only that sound for fifteen minutes.
- When you are finished, give thanks for the sounds in your life that are holy.
- Give thanks for your throat chakra, which allows you to tell the truth and to receive the truth. Give thanks for your voice, which is unique to you and only you.
- Bring this meditation into your daily spiritual practice and make your mantra "As I sound 'om,' I cocreate my life."

27. THE THIRD-EYE CHAKRA: THE INNER SIGHT CENTER

The inner sight chakra is located between the eyes. It allows us to see our illusions. Examine your motives and your dreams. Be sure to envision all you want in your life. Be certain that you are giving all you can to life.

The inner eye chakra, or third-eye chakra, is located in the middle of the forehead between the physical eyes and is part of the upper chakra system on the Path of Liberation. It allows us to see patterns in the world around us. It also allows us to see our illusions, which keep us from further growth on our path.

The inner eye chakra is the seat of clairvoyance, the ability to see the unseen. Other psychic abilities also reside here: clairaudience, the ability to hear what others cannot; clairsentience, the ability to be conscious of what is not obvious through either an "inner knowing" or a "feeling." The inner sight chakra is a part of our intuitive perceptual system. It helps us see, hear, feel, and become conscious. It helps us to function in the world on a deeper level than the cognitive. This center also deals with abstract thinking and visions. Here we sense most the presence of our spirit guides.

This chakra gives us the right to see with our inner eye the truth behind all that happens. Its color is indigo.

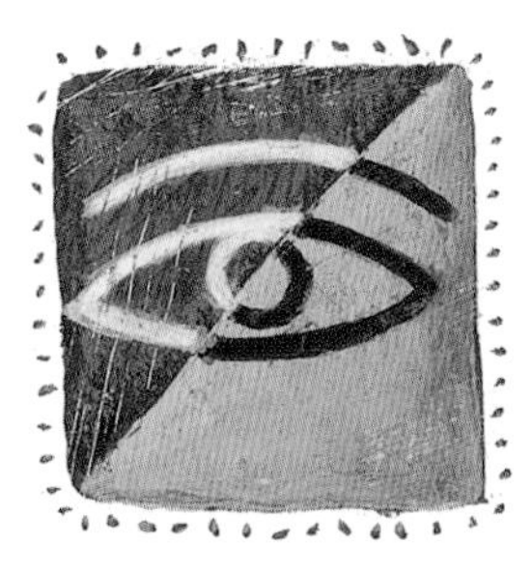

Within this archetype are two opposing forces, clear sight and blindness. Insight is a wonderful thing to have. It offers us a true picture of what is happening at any given time. But it is entirely possible to have too much insight. At the wrong times, insight without wisdom hurts us. Sometimes we are given a vision of what will happen or of what is happening that is not visible to others. We may have some psychic ability. We need all of our wisdom to decide who to tell and when to tell what we have seen.

Insight is also a deep knowing, a "gut feeling" or a "hunch." It includes sensing things and the whole realm of imagination.

At the other end of the spectrum is blindness. There are many degrees of blindness. We may be dim, dull, or shortsighted. We may have blurred vision. We may have distorted vision. We are often afraid to see what is right in front of us. We are afraid to see with our inner vision, and at times, we are most afraid to share what we know.

If we live too long at this end of the continuum we may not reach our spiritual goals. Move over toward the middle and toward the other end where you are not blind to the gifts you have been given. The gifts of your soul.

WHEN YOU DRAW THIS CARD you are being asked to tune in to your innermost heart's desires.

If the card is UPRIGHT, you have good insight into others. Be certain now that you also look into your own heart and see what is the truth.

If the card is REVERSED, you may be feeling dull right now in your life. Do the psychological and spiritual work necessary to gain insight into the situation.

EXERCISE: Wear the color indigo (a deep violet-blue) when you can for the next week and burn an indigo candle each day for seven days as you ask for help in this area.

AFFIRM with feeling: "My inner visions match my outward life. I create and manifest what I desire. I deserve good things in my life."

INNER SIGHT CHAKRA MEDITATION

- Move into a meditative position as you relax your body and relax your mind. Do not think. Only be still and receptive.
- Put the middle finger of your dominant hand in the middle of your forehead, over your third-eye chakra, while you do this meditation.
- Think of the color purple.
- On that color purple, print in large gold letters this affirmation: "I,[your name], have all the [time, money, health, abundance, love, energy] I want or could want in order to accomplish my soul's highest purpose."
- Then make an inner picture (or feeling or knowing) of what you want more than anything else in the whole world. Picture it in all detail. When the picture is complete, say: "It is done. Thanks be to God."

28. THE CROWN CHAKRA: COSMIC CONSCIOUSNESS

Get in touch with your Higher Self. Ask to become aligned with that self. Flow with the oneness of the Universe.

The crown chakra is the last of the spiritual chakras. It is the highest we can go spiritually and its symbol is the mandala. The crown chakra is at the top of the head, and circulates all around the top of the head. Its color is white, purple, and gold, and it is shaped like a radiant mandala, in all the colors of the rainbow spectrum.

From the crown chakra comes cosmic awareness and total freedom. The crown chakra gives us permission and the ability to know and understand what concerns us. Few people operate at this highest level, though we all aspire to it. The ways in which we are open to the connection of our Higher Self and how we use our imagination are functions of the crown. When this level of consciousness is activated, we are totally in alignment with our Higher Self. We become ascended masters at this level. We have mastered all of our karmic lessons.

When we do work with the crown chakra, we must also do work with the bubbling spring, which is on the bottoms of the feet, palms of the hands, and on the knees. When we are involved in healing, we need to pay attention to the palms, knees, ankles, and feet. This also grounds us to the earth and prevents light-headedness.

Within this archetype are two opposing forces, oneness and duality. Oneness is the highest spiritual concept we know and is worked for excessively and longingly by all spiritual seekers. When we live in the knowledge that there is no separation between God and the Universe, all living things included, there is a seamless quality to our daily lives.

However, human nature and our life on earth being what they are, the oneness we seek usually eludes us. It may occur in those "peak moments" when we are in tune with Nature or in flow with ourselves or in moments of intimacy with other living things. But we don't seem to be able to stay there. Nor should we. Our soul evolves through our earthly life.

We seem to have a basic nature that is dualistic. It wasn't just the philosopher Descartes who split us up. We are split by our very existence on earth. We are human beings trying to be spiritual. We are spiritual beings trying to be human. We feel as if we don't fully belong in either the spirit world or the human world. If we are to be psychologically and spiritually healthy, we must accept our human nature for what it is; while at the same time, we continue to seek the perfection of oneness.

WHEN YOU DRAW THIS CARD you are being asked to get in touch with your Higher Self.

When the card is UPRIGHT, you are on the right track with your spiritual intentions. Learn to become more practical.

When the card is REVERSED, you may be living too often in the state of duality, split off from your spiritual roots.

EXERCISE: In your meditations, visualize the color purple surrounding the top of your head. Burn a purple candle daily for the next week as you ask to be aligned with the will of the One.

AFFIRM with feeling: "I am aligned and in tune with my Higher Self and I express that self in all my business."

CROWN CHAKRA MEDITATION

- Draw a mandala. The mandala, you remember, is a symbol for Soul or God.
- It is also a symbol for the crown chakra. Make your mandala as beautiful as you can.
- Create it in all the colors of the rainbow. You can use markers, paints, pencils.
- When your mandala is finished, sit down with it in front of you and meditatively enter your mandala. Do not think. Do not speak. Just be with God. Remember the words "Be still and know I am with you."